ENJOYING YOUR TWILIGHT YEARS

Wisdom and insight from a Christian perspective as you prepare to retire with pleasure and fulfillment

Published 2023 by Terry J Boyle
Copyright Terry John Boyle 2023

Unless otherwise noted, all scripture quotations are from the Holy Bible,
New King James Version Copyright 1979, 1980, 1982
By Thomas Nelson, Inc.

Words in capitals, or bold or italics are the emphasis of the author
Terry Boyle terryjohnboyle@bigpond.com

Cover and typeset by Carl Butel at Deep Image
carl@deepimage.net.au

Cataloging-in-Publication data is available from the
National Library of Australia

ISBN 978-0-646-87786-0
eBook ISBN 978-0-646-87791-4

ACKNOWLEDGMENTS

I would like to thank my wife Caroline for her wonderful love and support over the years and for her chapter on "Aging" from a Woman's Perspective. Also our children Amanda, Felicity, Andrew, Sharon, and their spouses and children.

To our daughter Amanda for her encouragement, wisdom, insight, and input into the book, together with her husband Carl for the brilliant cover design, internal page layout, and getting this book ready to publish.

For my son Andrew, who is a Baptist minister, for his incredible wisdom, timely suggestions, proofreading, and adjustments to the book before printing.

To Dr Robert Easton for taking the time to read the manuscript and for his supportive input and gratifying foreword.

To those leaders, ministers, churches, friends, and relatives that have all impacted my life in so many different ways.

To the churches where we have been pastoring in some capacity in Melbourne, Port Moresby, Lismore, and Brisbane.

To the Churches on the Gold Coast where we have been fellowshipping in recent times.

To all those leaders and Christians on the Mission Field in Papua New Guinea.

To A2A as an organization for its leadership and inspiration over many years. Especially, Phillip Mutzelburg for his time to read the draft and endorse the book.

We are now enjoying our twilight years retired on the Gold Coast, in Queensland, Australia.

CONTENTS

ENJOYING YOUR TWILIGHT YEARS

FOREWORD

By Dr Robert Easton

MBBS, D Obst RCOG (retired)

It seems a lifetime ago that I first met Terry in Melbourne, Victoria. At the time I was at the beginning of my medical career which was going to span over 40 years in general practice. Terry was also at the beginning of a lifelong Christian ministry. He spent 21 years as the lead pastor in a successful church and also pioneered a Bible College in PNG. Strangely in our retirement years, our paths have once again crossed in a different state (Queensland) and a different church.

Terry asked me a short time ago if I would consider writing a foreword for this book. Having read the transcript I was most impressed with his practical and Godly approach to this challenging time of life which we all must eventually face.

While many people transition into this new stage of their lives in a relatively healthy manner, there are some who struggle. It is not always easy to deal with what can feel like a significant loss in one's life. The perceived loss of position, purpose, and relevance can at times weigh heavily on some.

In Chapter 9, titled **'How much does God love you?'** I believe Terry touched on a vital truth. God loves us not because of what we do or who we are. He loves us because of who He is! We are His sons and daughters! None of us are irrelevant no matter what stage of life we are in.

I pray that as you read this book the God of love will reveal Himself to you if you don't already know Him.

Dr Robert Easton

I hereby endorse this book...

From the very first lines of the first chapter, I knew this book by Terry Boyle was going to keep my attention. Being well into my twilight years I found chapter after chapter addressed the issues which are the subject of many coffee discussions with friends.

The simple but deeply profound way he untangles some of the complex questions of the senior years will position the reader to navigate their twilight years with increased expectation. As a result, they will be filled with peace, joy, and a sense of new adventures.

It will also be gold for younger readers to alert them to some of the pitfalls of not planning ahead.

Terry's book should be compulsory reading for everyone who wants to attain the quality of life God intends us all to enjoy.

Phillip Mutzelburg
Pastor Emeritus, Founder of Willow Creek Australia,
Founder of Acts 2 Alliance.

INTRODUCTION

I do not feel any older. That is until I look in the mirror and compare what I see with the pictures in our old photo albums. Then I think, *"Oh my goodness, what happened?"* Unfortunately, the weathering decades are not so kind to our appearance and physical capabilities.

Staying fit and healthy and feeling your best is important at any age. When I was younger, I never thought about getting old. Like many young people, I felt invincible and loved to play various sports to keep myself strong and agile.

But the reality is, as we grow older, we face several life changes. They vary for different people but might include career changes, retirement transition, children leaving home, losing a loved one, and physical and health challenges.

However, for me, the prospect of getting older is daunting. Completely out of my control; I can face it in fear or faith. I can choose to dwell on the negatives or the positives. Over the years, I have discovered that if I approach aging positively, it is not all doom and gloom and can be quite enjoyable.

As a retired pastor and missionary, I look through the lens of a Christian perspective. Despite the physical limitations we all experience as we grow older, our attitude is paramount. *"For the joy of the Lord is your strength"* – Nehemiah 8:10. There is nothing like a good dose of joy to help us through our twilight years!

I have never visited so many coffee shops and drunk so much caffeine as I do now. Probably not great for my waistline, but it gives me immense joy to be with my wife or friends having fellowship and a good laugh — even if we are inclined to tell the same stories and jokes repeatedly.

A few years ago, I wrote a book, **'Unlocking Your Purpose'**, about keys to discovering your God-given purpose in life. This was more for younger people with aspirations of leadership and ministry. Throughout Unlocking Your Purpose, I mixed sound biblical principles with experiences and memoirs I had encountered over many years in ministry. I was in retirement mode while writing and still finding fulfillment in the part-time activities of Bible College lecturing, preaching, and mentoring.

However, as the years have progressed, I now find myself entering the twilight years of my life. This is proving to be a testing time, with some frustrations I will address. Nevertheless, I pray that my vulnerability and sharing what I have learned will encourage and help you prepare for peaceful and pleasant "twilighting".

I understand that most people struggle with getting older. But not everyone responds the same. They either groan and moan or take a lighter note, saying (tongue in cheek), *"Oh, the joys of getting older"*.

I don't have all the answers, but I wanted to write this book to share some keys I have discovered that will hopefully help you to enjoy (rather than endure) the twilight years of your life.

Chapter 1

Coming to grips with your frustrations

As I enter my twilight years, it has been a time of frustration and joy, with many challenges. Honestly, it often feels like I live in slow motion compared to being in my prime.

There are noticeable external changes. For example, we face differences in our appearance, and our lack of flexibility and freedom of mobility limits our physical abilities. Recently while visiting our youngest daughter Sharon and her husband, Jeremie, I asked Sharon, *"Have you noticed how slow your mother is getting lately?"* To which she answered, *"So are you, Dad"*.

Yes, aging can be a frustrating time, but something we need to come to grips with. There are also more subtle internal adjustments, such as the emotional stress we experience when dealing with situations we cannot control. And to add insult to injury, we feel annoyed or upset with ourselves for being unable to handle something or someone.

The reason behind our frustration can be complicated. Some signs are fairly obvious, like when we feel anxious or on edge, we can become angry, and even lose our temper. We can feel overwhelmed, give up on certain tasks, and have trouble sleeping or eating. Some in their twilight years even turn to substances to cope (alcohol, nicotine, drugs).

Thankfully, there are healthier ways to deal with your frustrations. For example, you can talk to someone who can help you. And importantly, you can accept what you cannot change, and change what you can to relieve your stress levels. I will describe this in more detail as you read through these chapters.

An active lifestyle

Like myself, you may have been active in your working life. I have always been on the move doing something, going somewhere, my wife would often say, *"Just chill out and relax."*

I reflect on my exciting and adventurous years on the mission field, planning church programs and planting new churches — the visions and dreams for ministry and the local church. All this seems like a fond but fading memory.

We may also feel forgotten and neglected. For example, I recently visited a church I pastored for many years. I was welcomed and greeted as a newcomer and duly presented with a visitors pack! The person was new to the church.

You know you are getting old when a pastor jokingly introduces you to someone as a couple who have been around forever, saying *"They use to be Noah's youth pastors"*.

Although you may be recognised and shown respect by some pastors and churches, you are usually no longer consulted for wisdom and advice. This can make you feel well and truly past your use-by date. I am sure some of you think that way, even though you still have a lot to give that can benefit leaders, communities, and families. Sadly, you begin to doubt your value and wonder what the future holds for you in your twilight years. I know this also applies to those in the workforce.

'Festering' sore of ageism

The above heading leads into an article in a recent 'The Seniors News'. It reads:

AGEISM is alive and well in Australian workplaces and its crushing older workers. Mature workers are first in line for involuntary redundancy and subjected to ageist workplace banter and language, including ageist jokes and derogatory comments about physical fitness, sense of humour and appearance. Many feel patronised, excluded, undervalued, and fearful, and belittled because of their age, and pushed out the door prematurely. It's like a heavy shadow that eats away at you. It festers inside. You might initially be angry but end up feeling defenseless and useless.

This sober article reveals the plight of aging workers. Of course, all these factors may not apply in every situation. Still, it shows the frustration of getting older in the workplace as we contemplate retirement. Some can't wait to retire, while others want to keep going and have no intention of retiring, provided they can keep their place in the workforce.

Trying to stay fit and healthy

I love to fish and play golf, but that also has its frustrations as we age. I played golf the other day with a young guy in his late teens. He whacked the ball a mile (like I did years ago). I now hit nowhere near that far, but I still enjoy the game — except when things go wrong as they did when I was playing recently.

My son-in-law Carl (also a big hitter) gave me a fancy new golf buggy to which I could attach an umbrella for respite from the intense heat. The first time I tried it out, a gust of wind blew the umbrella into a big pond covered in water weeds. I thought if I walked into the water, I could retrieve it. So, assuming it was only an inch deep, I stepped in and went down — all the way to my armpits! After the initial shock, I reached for the umbrella but struggled to get out. I was tangled up in the weeds! Eventually, I scrambled back onto the green, covered in pond scum, looking like a sniper from a war movie.

When I first retired, I would run some laps around a nearby oval and sprint from one end to the other. I would also take long walks in the bush and lift weights in the gym. I still do some walking, a little running, and smaller gym sessions. Occasionally I swim laps in our pool. As retirees, our health and well-being depend on regular exercise, we must keep exercising, even if it is just going for walks. I also kept active by lecturing in a Bible College for several years and volunteered one day a week with VMR (Volunteer Marine Rescue).

I have also found solace and joy in art, mainly by painting seascapes, landscapes, and some abstract art, which only requires a little physical energy. Also, I keep my brain active by using my computer, watching TV, and revisiting old hobbies, like playing the guitar. My wife Caroline is more interested in puzzles, Sudoku crosswords, using her iPad, and watching TV. As we age, we must all keep ourselves occupied doing something.

Caroline and I both love to go for drives. We are fortunate to live in a beautiful part of the world on the Gold Coast, and there are plenty of places to explore. Occasionally we make more extensive trips to other parts of Queensland and Australia. We love the fuel economy of our Toyota Rav4 Hybrid and want to make the most of it while we can still drive.

Others in their twilight years do all sorts of voluntary work. Some become involved in their church, participate in a Men's Shed, or join a Club. The important thing is to keep engaged and do something.

In his book 'Lifespan', Dr. David Sinclair talks about why we age and why we don't have to. He expounds on the concepts of healthspan (living a healthy, high-quality life to death) and lifespan. He deals with practical strategies to make your health span equal to your lifespan and how to make your lifespan long and vibrant. Otherwise, he says, what is the point of having a long lifespan if it does not match your healthspan? I think this thought could be challenged, depending on your situation.

Health issues

Unfortunately, I have encountered some unpleasant and frustrating health issues that limit my physical capacity to do all I want. Besides some skin cancers I had removed over the years, I have been in pretty good health until recently. I have had radiation treatment and hormone therapy for prostate cancer. At the time of writing, all the treatment results have been successful, and there is no sign of cancer. Praise God! But as a believer in healing through prayer, I ask the obvious question, why was I not healed in answer to prayer? Why did I need to undergo these unpleasant medical procedures, especially after seeing so many people healed during my ministry? I have also just started medication for 'Occasional Atrial Fibrillation' in the heart. But I thank God for medical science and the healing it brings to millions around the world.

My wife Caroline has had some health issues too. Not long after we retired, she had minor surgery for breast cancer in its early stages. More recently, she has had a hip replacement and a cataract removed from one eye. But she still swims and walks regularly. She loves to garden with some help from me. I now get someone in to mow the lawns for us.

Disability Carers

You might say we have been fortunate, as I know of others as they age who have either ended up with a disability themselves or have a partner or child with a disability. Some of them require the constant services of trained caregivers.

Jonathan Tromane, in his book 'The twilight years', gives a personal account of working as a caregiver in the Australian Health Care system. He shares his experiences caring for various people with a range of physical and mental disabilities. He describes the issues they cope with each day. He says, *"The world's population is aging thanks to advances in medicine. People are living longer; many, however, still contract various medical conditions in different stages of their lives".*

Older people also rely on medication. Some have strict dietary needs and require regular therapy or treatment for different ailments.

Intimacy and sex

Someone who knew I was writing this book asked me if I would consider including a section about intimacy and sex as we get older. My immediate reaction was that they should mind their own business, it is personal and private. But then I thought well maybe they have a point.

Our children wince if we talk about sex and usually say, *"Too much information"* or *"Gross"*. In other words, they become embarrassed. So at the risk of embarrassing ourselves and others, I ran a few thoughts past my wife to see if she would let me put it in print. If you are reading this, you will know she is okay with it.

We are just as intimate with each other now as we have been. We take every opportunity to show one another love and respect. We make time for plenty of cuddles, hugs, and kisses. They are just as important as ever, but not as passionate as when we were younger. This includes being together most of the time, like shopping, having coffee, and occasionally going out for lunch or dinner. We like to help one another and work together as a team regarding budgeting, housekeeping, gardening, and other chores. We do not like being apart as we enjoy each other's company. Like any couple, we are not perfect and may feel we need a bit of space or time out, which usually only lasts for a short period. Like all couples, there are seasons when we need to work on our relationship and make some compromises.

As we age, sex is just one part of a range of intimate experiences we seem to enjoy. We feel that, if anything, the quality of our sex has not diminished with age. It has just become less frequent. We have both enjoyed sex and still do if and when it happens. We are both satisfied with this area of our lives. Since my treatment for prostate cancer, our sex life has slowed considerably. Thankfully, the doctors could preserve my nerves in the prostate region enabling me to function sexually with the help of a prescribed tablet.

I have spoken to other men who have had this treatment and can no longer perform sexually. When I tell them my story, they envy me and say, "You're a lucky man". However, the doctors say this will eventually wear off with age. So I guess we will have to wait and see what happens. In the meantime, I hope to enjoy being a "lucky man".

The best medicine

The best medicine is to maintain your joy. The 'Mayo Clinic' says that laughter *"Improves your immune system, activates and improves your stress response, soothes tension, and improves your mood."* The Bible says, ***"A merry heart does good like a medicine,*** *but a broken spirit dries the bones.*" – Proverbs 17:22.

Most Australians have a good sense of humour. We all like to be around happy people. I used to think the *"How do you know when you are getting old jokes?"* were so funny (still do), but now most of them have become a stark reality, like the one *"When the old lady you help across the street happens to be your wife."*

The late Pastor Trevor Chandler had a great sense of humour. He often started his sermon with a good joke to lighten the atmosphere. He ended up writing a 'joke' book!

But now and then, you come across someone who seems to have lost their sense of humour. They have been hurt, disappointed, and become bitter. I was talking to a disillusioned elderly retired minister recently who plans to write a book on everything the church was doing wrong to hurt people. I feel it is far better to be a blessing than to be bitter. When life hands you a lemon, you know the old saying! – *"Make Lemonade."* Life is too short to hold grudges.

Psalm 32:11 encourages us to **"Be glad in the Lord and rejoice, you righteous; and shout for joy, all you upright in heart."** Although, of course, there are times when this will seem impossible. But we can always start by thanking God for so great a salvation.

Ministry and work limitations

For me, ministry opportunities seem to decrease with age, which is regrettably understandable. I heard one enthusiastic young pastor say recently from the pulpit, *"Who would want to go and see a 70-year-old Mick Jagger strut his stuff?"* It was not a reflection on the singer's talent so much as the inference that older people have little to offer the younger generation.

There may be an element of truth in this. However, having certain talents, years of experience, and success must account for something — not only in the ministry but also in the workplace. The input of some older people and mature ministers has personally helped and blessed me.

After being retired for several years, we were helping out in a church in Brisbane, where I was regularly on the preaching roster. This was a rewarding and enjoyable time. Although I was in retirement mode, we felt loved, accepted, and appreciated during that time and developed meaningful relationships in that church.

Slow down to de-stress

When we get older, our stress levels seem more fragile. I get uptight over little things much more quickly than I use to. I have learned to distance myself from those things that tend to put us under undue pressure, including toxic relationships. I know my limitations and only take on what I am comfortable with managing. This means slowing down and taking on fewer commitments and having more time to relax.

I only had a few ministry engagements last year: a Church Camp and a National Leaders Conference in Port Moresby, Papua New Guinea. My wife and I are currently mentoring Geoff and Joan Haase a lovely pastoral couple in Toowoomba. We also minister in their church from time to time. So we are well and truly in semi-retirement mode.

We are currently enjoying the freedom to visit several great churches on the Gold Coast. This is something you can not do when you are the senior pastor of the church you are responsible for. We are not looking for ministry but enjoy listening to others and fellowshipping with so many people that we already know in these churches.

Aging is a privilege

We must never regret getting older, it is a privilege that not everyone has. It brings a tear to my eye when I think of some that have passed on prematurely, and will never have the privilege of getting older. Yes, there may be struggles and setbacks as we age, but what a joy we have to see our children and grandchildren growing up.

I admit life is not all 'happy-clappy', but I have discovered how to make it more enjoyable despite the setbacks. That is why I wrote, *Enjoying Your Twilight Years*.

In the following chapters, I invite you to journey with me as I unpack strategies I have learned to help you face the twilight years of your life with pleasure and fulfillment.

Chapter 2

Prepare well ahead of time

The Boy Scout motto is a good one – 'Be Prepared'. We need to be prepared for the twilight years.

Why prepare early? The aging process and its impact will be guaranteed, whether or not we prepare for it. Therefore it is wise to prepare for our twilight years in advance to prevent impending disappointment or trouble later in life. If we do prepare well ahead, we are far less likely to go into panic mode, realising we are completely unprepared when the time comes.

This usually begins with planning for retirement. It is estimated that only 53% of Australians are ready for retirement. So it is more important than ever to start planning for your post-work years. For most people, it is a delicate balance between maintaining a lifestyle and saving for the future. Planning will give you some sense of financial security.

C. S. Lewis said, *"You can't go back and change the beginning, but you can start where you are and change the ending"*.

Making decisions

Retirement can be a jungle of decision-making. What sort of assets to invest in? How long will your money last? Will you be eligible for the age pension?

There are plenty of good books around to help you like the 'Retirement Planning Guide Book' by Wade Pfau, Ph.D. CFA. RICP. This book helps you navigate through the important decisions to prepare you for your best retirement. It gives you the detailed knowledge and understanding to make smart retirement decisions.

I have had some people, especially Pastors, scoff at the thought of retiring, which for some, I can understand. Maybe retirement is not for everyone. I know when I first retired I would say I was semi-retired. When you have a calling on your life you never seem to fully retire. I continued to do some ministry but was not responsible as the senior pastor for any particular church.

It is interesting to read in Numbers 8:25 that the priests who ran the Old Testament Tabernacle had to retire. *"At age 50, they must retire from their regular service and work no longer"*. Mind you I think living conditions would have been tough in those days. 50 seems far too young to retire, whereas today around 65 plus seems to be the acceptable age for retirement.

From a Christian perspective, we need to be led by the Lord, if we retire, as to when and how to retire. The timing needs to be right for each individual. This is a very personal thing, and everyone will have a different perspective on this subject.

Some founding pastors of churches have had the privilege of their church supporting them financially in some way after their retirement. This is usually for an agreed time. But there are not too many churches in a financial position to do that these days.

I have heard other Pastors and some Christians glibly say there is no need to plan for retirement as God will provide. I admire their faith but not their lack of wisdom. As a result, I have seen many retirees struggle especially from a financial point of view. Some pastors are vulnerable in this area as they seem to think that it is a lack of faith to prepare for their retirement and that God will provide for them anyway.

I make an exemption for those who live in third-world countries where there is little or no support from their churches or governments. They are dependent not only upon their faith, but also on family members, relatives, and friends for their ongoing support and provision. This was evident to us while living in PNG.

A Vision for the Future

The wisest man that ever lived, apart from Jesus, was King Solomon. His advice was to have a vision by planning for it. Proverbs 29:18. ***"Where there is no vision the people*** *perish,"* I think it is only wise to prepare ahead to make the twilight years become more enjoyable.

Many years ago we had the privilege of having the late Hal Oxley and his wife Jill in our home for lunch. He was a colonel in the Australian Army and a businessman before entering the ministry. Hal was a visionary and thrived on scriptures like the above, and expected everyone to have a vision for the future. During lunch, he turned to our daughter Felicity when she was doing her HSC and asked her what her vision was for the future, to which she replied, *"I wouldn't have a clue."* He was horrified to think she had no vision.

I might add Felicity ended up doing interior design at the University of Technology Sydney and worked for an architect for a time. Her love for gardening and plants caused her to later study horticulture and she is now managing a nursery. The point is that vision is often progressive and unfolds as we go.

Preparing a successor

If we have a vision for the future and we are going to retire we need to prepare a capable successor to replace us whether it be in the workforce or the church.

Father and son successions are often very successful. My brother-in-law Robert who owns a factory engineering business has turned 80 and at this stage is not planning to retire but will eventually hand over to his son Lucas.

Phillip and Mandy Mutzelburg handed over their A2A Catalyst Church in Ipswich to their son Carl and his wife

Jessica. This has been a great success.

I was fortunate enough to have my associates Rod and Margaret Dymock take over Centre Church in Lismore. They have recently handed over to Dave and Bernie Winter. All of these transitions have been successful and have maintained a vibrant vision for the future.

A proposal for you to consider

I realise that what I am about to propose may sound intimidating, and may not be a viable or affordable plan for you. You may be struggling to pay the rent or the mortgage and the bills at this stage in your life. You may be content to get a pension or some kind of government support in your retirement years.

My wife and I, have been fortunate enough, by the grace of God, to be in a position to plan for our retirement many years in advance. This is how we went about it. Hopefully, it will sow some seeds for you to contemplate and work on.

Create income streams and reduce your debt

To become financially independent, we started to plan to create some income streams to help us reduce our debt, hoping that by the time we retired, we would be debt free, and build financial security for our future.

We began by working hard and saving what we could. For most of our younger married lives, we were both working. So we had two income streams. During this time we were very careful with our spending and went without a lot of luxuries. We rented for the first five years of our married lives but saved hard to have enough deposit for our first home. We were able to buy a block of land and build in Melbourne with the help of a substantial loan from the bank.

Apart from the strategy just mentioned. People have successfully turned their creative talents and hobbies into income streams. I had a cousin who did photography as a hobby. He started off using his bathroom to develop negatives. Someone asked him to do their wedding. He did such a great job, word got around and because of the demand for his services, he started up his own business. He later became involved in printing high-class photographic material and magazines and as a result, became very wealthy. I'm sure you have heard similar stories.

Our daughter Amanda is a brilliant abstract artist who has the potential to turn her hobby into an income stream. She needs to become known for her work in such a competitive field. You can check out her work on Instagram "Amanda Butel Art".

Invest wisely

Some years later, we were fortunate enough to inherit some money from both our parents after they had passed on. The first thing we did with our first inheritance, was to clear our debt, by paying off our mortgage on the house we were living in at the time.

With the next inheritance, instead of spending our money on a new car or other things that we may have liked to have obtained at the time, we decided to make some investments for our retirement. We decided to invest in shares and real estate.

Well before receiving our inheritances, we had bought a package of CBA shares for $5.75 a share. The last time I looked they were somewhere between $90.00 to $100.00 a share. Of course, shares can be risky and fluctuate dramatically, which can be off-putting to some people. However, as a long-term investment, statistics show that if $10,000 was invested in 1992 into an ASX200 fund (representing the top 200 companies in the Australian Stock Exchange), it would be worth over $130,000 today. This is a compounding return of 9.8% per annum, far better than keeping the money in a savings account. So we have tried to stick to a handful of 'Blue Chip' shares, which history shows are usually more stable and reliable.

We also had enough deposit, together with a loan from the bank, for an investment house. For the first ten years, we had to be disciplined to pay off the loan, but over a while, it was paid off and we were able to repeat this process, ending up with another two investment houses. By the time we retired, they were all paid off. So this gave us an income stream from the rent, together with some dividends from shares.

Build up your superannuation

When we retired we did not have a lot of superannuation.

It became compulsory in Australia while we were on the mission field in PNG. So we did not have any super commence until we returned to work in Australia. But we were able to build up our Super to give us a little more financial security. So the little super we had by the time we retired gave us another potential income stream. However, our Superannuation alone would never have been enough to retire on, which is why we are grateful to have built up several other income streams in shares and property.

We read in Habakkuk 2:2 *"Write the vision and make it plain"* The inference is to plan well so you have something to follow. Using this principle we deliberately planned for our retirement. You may not have received an inheritance, or you may have had circumstances, or disasters that have led to a financial hardship that prevents you from being able to do much to prepare for the future. If that is the case I want to encourage you that it is never too late though to start thinking about budgeting and planning for your future retirement.

Keep on giving

We must not forget the principle of giving. The Bible encourages us to be generous when it comes to giving. We have tried to put this into practice throughout our married lives and know from experience it pays dividends.

> *"He who sows sparingly will also reap sparingly, and he who sows bountifully will also reap bountifully. So let each one give as he purposes in his heart, not grudgingly or of necessity; for*

God loves a cheerful giver. And God is able to
make all grace abound toward you, that you,
always having all sufficiency in all things, may
have an abundance for every good work".
– 2 Corinthians 9:6-8.

Not that we should think that just by giving we create an income stream without taking responsibility to earn an income. But as we can see by the above scripture, there is a blessing in giving.

People ask me who or what should we give to. Christians should give to their local church and also to credible organisations like 'Compassion' or 'Vision'. There are many others, but I would like to mention 'Destiny Rescue' because our daughter Amanda and her husband Carl both work for the organisation that primarily rescues children from the sex trafficing trade in several countries. As a family, they have spent three periods in Thailand volunteering for Destiny Rescue. The longest being almost a year.

Playtime for some

There is a saying 'Pay now and Play later' or 'Play now and Pay later'. The thought behind this is, if you 'Pay' now when you are young by working hard, saving, and investing for the future when you get older you can 'Play' by having a great time spending and having enough to do what you want to do. We worked on this principle.

I had always loved being around boats. As we neared retirement we had a bit of extra money, I said to my wife, *"I would love to buy a boat"*. Her less-than-enthusiastic, sarcastic reply, was, *"You can name it over my dead body"*. However, she eventually relented (a miracle).

Most people would be looking at Caravans. But, we ended up buying a second-hand Haines Hunter 7.1 meter Cruiser, it was a lovely boat with twin 150 H.P. motors. We had lots of wonderful adventures mainly cruising around the Gold Coast Broadwater. I think my wife ended up loving the boat more than I did.

I will never forget the time we took our son-in-law Carl and our grandson Bailey out overnight. We anchored in a lovely sheltered cove. They slept in a tent on the bank while my wife and I slept on the boat. Just after midnight, there was a loud thump and the boat lurched over on its side and I was thrown out of bed. We had not allowed for the low tide and we were high and dry leaning over on the beach. It was a lovely starry night, Carl got a big fire going for us so we could stay warm next to it on "camping" chairs in our sleeping bags. Carl later disappeared into the darkness and went off fishing. He came back with some of the biggest "Whiting" I've ever seen. In the morning as soon as we had cleaned the fish, the tide came back in, and we were floating again, we packed up, and off we went heading for home. After many years of enjoyment, we sold the boat.

Some Questions you should ask yourself

1. **Do I have a long-term plan of action?**

2. **What steps can I take now to prepare?**

3. **Am I prepared to commit to a plan?**

4. **What could stop me from moving ahead?**

5. **Who can I be accountable to for this plan?**

6. **How will I keep track of my progress?**

7. **What do I hope to achieve long term?**

No matter where you are at this stage in your life. I would still encourage you if you are in a position to start planning, then do so. You might be saying well it is too late for us to do that, we have little or no income stream to look forward to at this stage. Do not despair! We are fortunate enough in Australia to be able to fall back on the pension, and government assistance if we have no other source of income for retirement.

The one mistake you can not afford to make

We have been looking at preparing for retirement and the future. As much as we need to be diligent in doing this, the greatest mistake anyone can ever make in life is; NOT to prepare to meet God. You will eventually meet God. Are you prepared? If you died tonight and stood before God how would you feel?

Hopefully what I have shared will give you some insight and wisdom for a more enjoyable future as you prepare to retire and enter your twilight years.

Chapter 3

The key to your contentment

If only we could find contentment in our twilight years! What a huge difference that would make. Life would be so much more enjoyable. Is it possible? What could be the key for you?

Happiness depends upon good experiences whereas contentment is something we can have despite whatever state we may be in. Contentment is maintaining an inner peacefulness, gratitude, and satisfaction despite our circumstances.

I was ministering in India some years ago and turned on the TV where I was staying, and listened to some Guru speaking about how you could stay happy. His philosophy on happiness was based on trying to better your circumstances, and to keep smiling at all times no matter what was happening. This may be helpful but not what real contentment is in Christ. There are plenty of books written on contentment from a New Age point of view. But we need to stick to what we can glean from the bible.

Christian principles

There are some good books based on Christian principles. One such book is 'Chasing Contentment' by Eric Raymond. His theme is 'Trusting God in a discontented age'. He talks about recovering the lost art of contentment like it is something reserved for spiritual giants, but out of reach for the rest of us. He goes on to help us understand what biblical contentment is and how we all can discover how to have it.

Here is a good definition of contentment – *"It is finding inner joy in what we already have in our lives, and feeling or showing satisfaction with our possessions, status, or situation. It is being content without trying to find fulfillment in acquiring more material things".*

Contentment is about accepting people and things the way they are, and not dwelling on the way you wish they were. It's about keeping a positive attitude when things are difficult, or hard to understand, and why they are not fulfilling your expectations.

A worldly point of view

From a worldly point of view we are inclined to think if only we had more, we would be content. The more of everything, a better income, a better house, a better car, a better job, better health, and so the list goes on. We all want to do better, and there is nothing wrong with wanting to be blessed with more. After all, Jesus said **"I have come that you might have**

life and that you might have it more, abundantly" –
John 10:10.

But in our pursuit of wanting more, there seems to be a
fine line between coveting and envy. I once heard someone
say *"Covetousness wants what the other guy has; Envy is being angry
that the other guy has it".*

There seems to be a voice in our heads that tells us, we
need what THEY have, to be more acceptable, respectable,
and loveable. The Bible warns us that it is only going to harm
us, not help us if we become envious of others. ***"A sound
heart is life to the body, but envy is rottenness to the
bones"*** – Proverbs 14:30. It certainly seems that envy is not
a good thing for our health. It is something we can do without
and should avoid.

We also read in Ecclesiastes 4:10-13 ***"To envy others
is vanity and grasping for the wind."*** In other words,
there is no end to it. You cannot grasp or control the wind.
You no sooner get something better, than you want something
better again. Maybe it is the pressure we feel to be 'Keeping
up with the Joneses.' It goes on to say ***"Better is a handful
with quietness (tranquillity) than both hands full,
together with toil and grasping for the wind".*** The
implication is that it may be more beneficial at times to have
less. One handful with contentment rather than both handfuls
with trouble.

Godliness with contentment

The apostle Paul sums it up pretty well when addressing the

issue of those whose focus is on money, wealth, greed, and the pitfalls that go with it. ***"Now godliness with contentment is great gain"*** In other words, you are ahead, and doing well if you have both godliness and contentment.

Paul goes on to imply that if you are dependent on your wealth and possessions for contentment, you can not take them with you when you die. ***"We brought nothing into the world, and it is certain we can carry nothing out."*** – 1 Timothy 6:6-7.

Sure, it's nice to have plenty of stuff, but we can become so preoccupied with clutter, and material possessions, we lose sight of eternal values. What matters to God is our relationship with Him. This is our priority, together with our relationship to family and others.

The key to both natural and spiritual Contentment

How then can you find contentment in your twilight years? What is the key? I heard my son Andrew who is now a Baptist minister preach a great message on this subject. We find the answer in Philippians chapter 4 where it is thought that Paul is writing either in prison or under house arrest.

"Not that I speak in regard to need, for I have LEARNED in whatever state I am, to be content. I know how to be abased, and I know how to abound." – Philippians 4:11-12. The first thing we notice is that Paul is saying he has LEARNED how to be content in whatever state he is in. It is not natural for us to just be content, it is something we need to LEARN.

Several things the bible says in the context of Philippians Chapter 4, that we should learn-

1. *Learn to give thanks in all things*

2. *Learn to be satisfied with a little or a lot*

3. *Learn to survive your circumstances*

4. *Learn to rely on God's provision*

5. *Learn to help others in need*

However, the real KEY to CONTENTMENT is found in verse 13 *"I can do all things through Christ who strengthens me"*. So Paul is saying we need to be content with the Lord's graciousness for a peaceful life. He is saying he can go through anything God sets before him, for he knows the Lord will provide the strength he requires to complete the difficult trial he may be going through at the time. It is Christ who gives us the strength to cope with whatever state we are in.

Adapting when you are in the will of God

I think of the pokey old flat we rented, in Adelaide when we first got married and attended Bible College. But we were completely content. Then we moved to a tiny one-bedroom flat in Melbourne. But again we were content because we were in the will of God and He gave us the strength we needed for both situations, at that time in our lives.

We later spent six years on the mission field in Papua New

Guinea. The first year we were there we had no house. We moved around from 'leave-house' to 'leave-house' (house sitting) with our three children at the time - (our fourth one Sharon was born in PNG). This lasted for 12 months. It was for security reasons when people went away and wanted someone in to house sit.

Some house sits had animals to look after. In one house they had a lovely dog, a red setter which we had to check regularly for ticks. One day I thought I had found a tick, which I started to pull with a pair of tweezers. The dog glared at me and started yelping, I was pulling on one of the dog's nipples. But I stopped before any damage was done.

During this time it was not easy for us, and it tested our joy. But we were happy and content despite the circumstances, for we knew we were in the will of God, doing what we were called to do. We finally moved into a house that was built for us on the church property.

During this time God was pouring out His Spirit in a wonderful way. Hardly a week went by without someone being saved, healed, or delivered. We saw incredible growth in the church in Port Moresby. From around 120 to 500 plus over five years. We wouldn't trade that experience for anything.

When we finally returned to Australia we were asked to take over the senior role of a church in Lismore that was going through a difficult time. At first, we were reluctant but we grew to love the Church and Lismore as a city. We were able to bring stability to the church and Christian School the

Church was pioneering at the time. We ended up staying there for 21 years.

In short, we have discovered that if you are in the will of God and obedient to His calling upon your life, He will give you the strength to be content, wherever you are, and in whatever state you are in at the time.

Do not be anxious – Pray!

Paul gives more insight into contentment earlier in Philippians 4:6-7. *"Be anxious for nothing, but in everything by prayer and supplication, with thanksgiving, let your requests be made known to God; and the peace of God, which surpasses all understanding, will guard your hearts and minds through Christ Jesus"*. We should never underestimate the power of prayer. When we become anxious, we should bring it to God in prayer. It is amazing how the peace of God disperses our anxiety, even when we are going through things we do not understand.

As you enter into your twilight years, the real secret to contentment is found in Christ who strengthens you and enables you to go through all things, no matter whatever state you find yourself to be in. You can therefore enjoy the twilight years more if you embrace and apply this truth.

Chapter 4

Watch your attitude

Many times since retiring I have had to work hard on watching my attitude. My wife and I often remind each other to watch our attitude if we start to focus on negative things. It is so easy for us to become critical, cynical and judgemental. But it robs us of our joy and our ability to be a blessing to others.

When we visit churches, having been a senior pastor, it is easy to see things we have been guilty of being repeated or something questionable which affects our attitude towards the leader, or the church. We have to remember that we have probably been there and done that ourselves at some stage.

Over the years we develop attitudes about certain things that influence our beliefs, on not only how churches should function – but also on other things like politics, sports, careers, and the workplace. Usually, these attitudes stay with us because of our background and upbringing by our parents, teachers, and community leaders. We often have strong opinions because of the things we have been taught. So the attitudes that we develop may be a result of our environment, and the people that influence our lives, either positively or negatively.

Improve your health with positive thinking

Here is a copy of a paper on 'Positive Thinking' by the Mayo Clinic Staff –

Positive thinking helps with stress management and can improve your health. Researchers continue to explore the effects of positive thinking and optimism on health and say some of the main benefits are – Lower rates of depression, distress, pain and illnesses, and also better coping skills in stressful situations.

Is your glass half empty or half full? How you answer this age-old question about positive thinking may affect your outlook on life, your attitude toward yourself, and whether you are optimistic or pessimistic, and it may even affect your health. If you tend to be pessimistic, do not despair – you can still learn positive thinking skills. Use positive affirmations, focus on the best outcomes and not the worst, concentrate on the present moment and not the too-distant future, and do something to help others. Whenever possible, surround yourself with positive people. Some relationships will be more beneficial than others.

Positive thinking does not mean that you ignore unpleasant situations in life. However, it means you approach them in a more positive and productive way, enabling you to better control your reactions and decisions.

How do you react to a problem?

How you react to a problem can quickly reveal your attitude. One of my sons-in-law, Greg, had at one stage on his computer the caption, *'The problem is not the problem, the problem is your attitude toward the problem'*. How true that is! How we react is key to how we handle the problem. Some say 10% of your life involves problems and 90% is on how you handle them.

After I preached one morning a lady came up to me and said, *"Your sermon was good but simple"*. Guess what I dwelt on? Yes, the word 'simple'. My immediate reaction was not good. I thought she was telling me I was a simple preacher. Then I remembered what we had been taught about preaching in Bible College, 'KISS' the people, 'Keep It Simple Stupid'. (So everyone can understand what you are saying). I stopped reacting and took it as a backhanded compliment.

Defining an attitude

The dictionary defines attitude as – 'the way we think, feel and act about a given situation'. Psychologists define attitudes as *'A learned tendency to evaluate things in a certain way, including evaluations of people, issues, objects, or events'*. Attitudes are often the result of our experiences. They can have a powerful influence over behaviour and affect how people act in various situations.

There are 3 main components to your attitudes –

1. **Your Thinking** – Thoughts and beliefs about a particular subject.

2. **Your Feelings** – On a subject, person, issue or event, as to how they may make you feel.

3. **Your Behaviour** – How an attitude influences your reaction or behaviour

Unity for the sake of the gospel

When it comes to attending church in the twilight years of our lives we have to be careful that we maintain a good attitude, despite things we may not like. We read where Paul says in Philippians 1:27 *"...that you stand fast in one spirit, with one mind, striving together for the faith of the gospel."*

We, therefore need to see the bigger picture. We should be supportive of one another for the sake of the gospel. If we are to impact our community for Christ they will need to see and hear us being positive. Christians and Non-Christians will not want to hang around people with negative attitudes.

In Philippians 2:3-4 Paul admonishes us to *"Let nothing be done through selfish ambition or conceit, but in lowliness of mind let each esteem others better than himself. Let each of you look out not only for his own interests but also for the interest of others"*. We should try and remain humble and praise others and take an interest in their vision and ministry.

Then in verses 14-15, we read *"Do all things without complaining or disputing, that you may become blameless and harmless, children of God without fault in the midst of a crooked and perverse generation, among whom you shine as lights in the world".*

So we need to watch our attitudes when we do church for the sake of the gospel, as the world is watching ready to pick on our faults.

Attitudes are contagious

Our attitudes are contagious and they affect others. Our negative attitudes have a negative effect, just as our positive attitudes have a positive effect. If our attitudes are contagious, let me ask you this question, "Is your attitude worth catching?" If it is positive and helpful it is certainly worth catching.

We worked with the late John Pasterkamp in Port Moresby, PNG. John had a contagious attitude. He was warm and friendly, and always pleased to see you. He was complimentary, and positive and made you feel valued and loved. His attitude was so contagious that you wanted to be like him.

This reminds me of the Apostle Paul, who encouraged others to imitate him, or more pointedly, to imitate him as he imitated Christ. Like it or not our behaviour both good and bad will influence others. Sure, Paul wasn't perfect – he had his challenges, particularly in various personal conflicts with other ministers and leaders. However, Paul worked on this area and strived to become more and more like Christ throughout his life.

Last-day attitudes in the world

I think we are inclined to grow up developing bad or negative attitudes in this fallen world we live in today.

In 2 Timothy 3:1-5, we have a description of what kind of attitudes and behaviours (as they usually go together) we can expect in these last days. I will take the liberty of paraphrasing this scripture. *"In the last days, people will love themselves, money, and pleasure more than God. They will be disobedient to their parents, unthankful, unholy, unloving, and unforgiving. Also proud, having a form of godliness but denying its power."*

Yes, there are a host of bad attitudes in that lot. We can see all these things happening around us today. We as Christians should be as lights displaying positive attitudes that counteract these negative ones.

When I was a boy I had a cousin living nearby. One Sunday I called in to see if he wanted to come with me to Sunday school. His father came to the door and said to me, "He is not going with you, we do not believe in that rubbish, it is not for us. I suspect his attitude may have been a result of a bad experience with some Christians or Christianity.

Today, many react to the gospel in different ways. Some respond in faith, while others display bad attitudes toward the gospel. Our job is to sow seed knowing that some will fall on good ground and reap a harvest.

Unacceptable payback attitudes

There was a time when Jesus had to correct the bad attitude of His disciples who wanted to destroy a Samaritan village for not receiving them. James and John said to Jesus, *"Do you want us to call down fire from heaven and consume them, just as Elijah did?"* But Jesus rebuked them and said *"You do not know what manner of spirit you are of, for the Son of man came to save men's lives not destroy them"* – Luke 9:51-56. The disciples felt it was payback time. That kind of judgemental, attitude is not Christlike.

Jesus came to demonstrate love, forgiveness and grace. We may not go to that extreme with our attitude, but we may feel like it, especially when we have been rejected, offended, or hurt in some way.

A good attitude releases faith

On the other hand, a good attitude can release faith. I find it so easy to preach and get a positive response in PNG mainly due to the attitude of the people which is usually full of faith and expectancy.

We see this in the attitude of two blind men when Jesus asked them *"Do you believe I can do this?"* They answered, *"Yes, Lord"*. They displayed a positive attitude that released faith, despite being blind. Jesus touched their eyes saying *"According to your faith let it be to you."* – Matthew 8:28-29. A good positive attitude seems to release faith for healing, miracles, and the blessing of God.

You can change your attitude

Attitudes are not permanent. You can change your attitude. We may be locked into a negative attitude or mindset about something, and believe we are still in the will of God. We can even in our mind justify the attitude we have developed even though it is not right.

We read in Acts 10:9-16 that there was a time when Peter was praying and became hungry, and wanted to eat. He fell into a trance and saw in the spirit God let down a sheet full of all kinds of animals. The Lord said to Peter *"Rise, Peter, kill and eat."* Peter refused and said, *"No Lord for I have never eaten anything common or unclean."* Imagine saying no to the Lord.

Peter justified his attitude because of his traditional teaching. But God was trying to change his attitude, to prepare him to take the gospel to the Gentiles, who were traditionally thought to be unclean. The Lord responded to Peter's 'no attitude' by saying *"What God has cleansed you must not call common."*

Peter eventually got the message and went and preached the gospel to the Gentiles. Surely there is a lesson here for all of us. Not to be quick to try and justify a wrong attitude because of our traditional thinking, background, or negative experiences in life. May we be willing to change our attitude to conform to the will of God!

Some practical tips

Yes, you can change your attitude. Here are some practical tips you need to consider –

1. Take responsibility for your attitude

2. Stop blaming others for your attitude

3. Forgive others who may have affected you

4. Try and avoid negative people and situations

5. Let go of unrealistic expectations

If you are a Christian, you should be quick to try and make all your negative experiences a matter of prayer, commit them to the Lord, and be willing to change your attitude and start rejoicing. *"Rejoice in the Lord, always, again I say, rejoice."* – Philippians 4:4.

This is easier said than done. But if we can rejoice in the Lord. Not for everything that happens in life, but in the Lord, who gives us inner peace, it will make our twilight years much more enjoyable.

As we grow older, may God help us NOT to become like those in the movie, 'Grumpy Old Men' (and women) and may He give us the grace to keep a watch over our attitude at all times.

Chapter 5

Value your relationships

What value do you put on your relationships? Are they precious and worth developing, fostering, and keeping for life?

Because of the fragility, and the volitivity of human nature, we usually only have a limited number of good relationships that we value throughout our lifetime.

We live in a broken world and relationships can become very fragile and subject to change at the drop of a hat. Many of us have experienced dysfunctional, damaged, and broken relationships. Hopefully, many of those relationships can be healed and restored by the grace of God. If not, it may be best to move on and commence new and more meaningful relationships. We were designed by God to develop good relationships.

The value of good relationships

Christianity is all about relationships. Our relationship with God, with our family, with our church, with our neighbours, with our community, and with the world.

When I was pastoring, I would have to be naive to think the only reason people came to our church was because of my leadership and preaching. That may be true for some, but the majority came because of the relationships they had developed with one another.

As we enter the twilight years, we know how valuable and important loving fulfilling relationships are, especially with our family and friends.

I was fortunate enough to have had a great relationship with my parents, my sister Lyn, and my relatives. As parents, we have also had a wonderful rapport with our own four children, who we love dearly, and our grandchildren.

I never grew up having a relationship with my grandparents as they were both deceased. Being a grandparent with grandchildren is now one of the highlights of my life. It was an area of my life I had missed out on. However, in a way, I'm making up for it, as we have fourteen grandchildren. We value our relationship with them and love them all to bits.

Relationship skills

In her book *Connect with Others and Yourself* Mary K. Tatum, MS, LMHC states that *"Relationship skills and social skills are referred to as "skills" for a reason – they require learning, practice, and refinement, the limited engagement is leaving many of us feeling out of practice with these skills, and disconnection is leading to emotions filled with fear, stress, anxiety, and depression".*

Most relationships require us to refine our skills to be able to be flexible and adjustable in our relationships. Everybody is different and we have to realise that it takes skill to relate to different people and their personalities and interests.

We can not afford to pre-judge or determine how we think a relationship is going to develop. We may have vastly different opinions about things and we should not expect that everybody is going to think the same way we do.

A relationship drought today

Professor Parkinson and Doctor Jensen put out a study paper with the title *A relationship drought today.* We are familiar with droughts in Australia. However, this study was done to gauge the result of the isolation effects of Covid-19. It showed how people stopped coming to church, how Church became more digital, with live streaming, and how this affected relationships. People became disconnected. There was an increase in loneliness among the elderly. People became desperate to develop meaningful face-to-face relationships. Many other things were also listed as a part of this study that had affected our relationships today.

During the Covid-19 lockdowns in our area, we stayed home and watched a smorgasbord of online churches. One of our many favourites was Legana Christian Church in

Tasmania and the brilliant teaching of Pastor Dr. Andrew Corbett. (We still tune in at times).

Hopefully, most of that has passed, as Covid-19 restrictions have now been lifted, and face-to-face relationships are being restored and developed once again. We are trying to settle down again. We are inclined to visit several churches in our area, as I have mentioned this is something you can not do when you are the senior pastor and responsible for your church. The ones we visit mainly are namely City on a Hill Church at Maudsland (Apostolic), Highway Church Ormeau (ACC), Authentic Church Meadowbrook (AOG), and Southport Church of Christ. We relate to people in all these churches.

Relational Value

There is a term known as 'relational value'. People may value relationships differently. No one thinks of their relationship with a colleague as highly as their friendship with a childhood friend, partner, or spouse. The value that each person perceives out of a relationship is called the 'relational value'.

Over the years I have worked with people in a 'relational value' capacity. You may have had the same experience in your workplace where you were dealing with people who have a different 'relational value' with you than what you have had with your spouse and family. But they are still valuable and meaningful relationships.

Having been in the ministry for many years we have many relationships with people we value with our roots going back to Life Ministry Church, Melbourne. Many leaders and Christians in PNG. After 21 years in Lismore, Centre Church Lismore, Meadowbrook Christian Church, Brisbane. Many ministers and leaders of the A2A (Acts 2 Alliance) movement. There are many other relationships we value, but if I start mentioning individual names, I will go on forever.

Although, I must mention I have still maintained a good relationship with Gary Parsons, a boyhood friend, who became our best man at our wedding, even though we may have different values, and have been separated by distance. We usually meet up with Gary and Gaye once a year when they come up from Victoria to Queensland to escape the Victorian winter.

Our local fish and chip shop

Our local fish and chip shop was run by a happy-go-lucky couple from the Philippines. They were always pleased to see you and they would chat and make you feel welcome. They had a nice waiting area with the latest newspapers and magazines to put people at ease. They developed valuable relationships with their customers, but not the same 'relational value' as your own family. They also served up great fish and chips! However, they sold out to a Chinese couple who did away with the nice waiting area, including all the newspapers and magazines. They are a serious couple who do not have the same knack for making you feel all that welcome. Unfortunately, they seem to have no sense of humour and have made little effort to develop relationships with their customers. And the fish and chips are nowhere near the same standard as before. I feel, 'the writing is on the wall', and that it is only a matter of time before the business fails. So we see how important it is to maintain good relationships. I believe there are some valuable lessons here to be learned in regard to the value of relationships for all pastors, and churches.

Relationships through church

The Church should be an ideal place to develop meaningful relationships. We all like a warm welcome, but people need more than just the usual greeting in the foyer like "Hello and Welcome or 'Nice to see you', or a parting goodbye like 'Have a great week' as you walk out.

Most churches these days make provision for a coffee and something to eat immediately after the service. It may not be for everyone, but it is a great opportunity to get to know someone and begin to develop ongoing relationships.

It is always good to have an open altar to pray for people who need prayer and support. This allows you the opportunity to make contacts that may need following up.

Meaningful relationships are the foundation of true happiness and living a full and fruitful life. They provide us with friends and family to share our life with. There are usually plenty of laughs and joy that give us a full and pleasurable lifestyle. The key elements of any meaningful relationship will include trust, loyalty, faith, faithfulness, honesty, mutual interests, and communication.

Psychotherapist Dr. Jamie Brodarick Ph.D. who is a licensed

Marriage and Family therapist says *"A healthy relationship allows the ability to balance being a strong individual with deep intimacy."* Healthy relationships are so important for married couples and the family unit.

God is relational

God himself shows us that He is relational, and desires to relate to us. In Genesis 2:26-28, We see how relational God is within the Trinity (Father, Son, and Holy Spirit), we have words like US, OUR, and THEM. Then, God said, ***"Let US create man in OUR image and OUR LIKENESS".*** He places man in the Garden of Eden (Adam and Eve) and gives them instructions on how to tend the garden. He visits them and relates to them. ***"And they heard the sound of the Lord God walking in the garden in the cool of the day"... "Then the Lord God called to Adam and said to him, "Where are you?"*** – Genesis 3:8-9.

This reference was after they had sinned by disobeying God. They were hiding because they were embarrassed to face God. Just like we are when we know we have sinned. So as a result sin entered the human race which separated us from God. But God eventually sent His Son Jesus so that we could be reconciled to God. He longs for a relationship with us. That includes you and me.

He also said in Genesis ***"That it is not good for a man to be alone."*** We are designed and created by God not to be alone, but to be relational, just like God.

Reconciliation before revival

I was invited to speak at a leadership conference in Port Moresby last year with Barry Winton, a fellow minister. They told us the theme would be 'Reconciliation for the New Wine.' I thought what a strange theme for a conference. But then after hearing of many issues that had caused broken relationships and divisions, I understood that there was a great need for leaders and people to be reconciled for the new wine of the Holy Spirit to flow again. They were desperate for a fresh move of the Spirit. By the grace of God, we saw many reconciled and healed from hurts and disappointments. We felt like our mission was accomplished and things were set in place for the new wine to flow again.

We loved our time in Papua New Guinea when we lived there on the mission field. The people are so easy to relate to and open to the gospel, and they long for meaningful relationships.

First Nations People

First Nations Australians are often referred to as Aboriginal and Torres Strait Islander peoples. But there is a significant diversity within these two groups. There is a wide range of cultures and languages across mainland Australia and throughout the Torres Strait.

We have been to Thursday Island in the Torres Strait and have found that many First Nations people are very open to and have embraced the gospel. Although they enjoy their own culture they do long for a more amicable relationship with all Australians.

Because of our time in PNG, we were appalled at the way some foreigners looked down on and treated the nationals. We see some Australians doing that to some degree in Australia in their attitude toward First Nations peoples. It needs to be something we should be aware of especially as we age. We should show more respect and honour to our First Nations peoples. After all, we are all one through the blood of Christ.

People are desperate for loving relationships

We have listened to Doctor Phil on TV interview several women, who through searching for love on the Internet had gone into relationships, only to be ripped off by men wanting money. They were so desperate, that even when Doctor Phil was able to prove that they had been conned, they were still in denial and did not want to believe the truth.

I was speaking to a Christian man, who had been a farmer. He had recently lost his wife and was very lonely. He said that they had planned to travel around Australia. Then he said he was still planning to do that, and that he would take his wife with him. He was going to sit her ashes in an urn on the dashboard of his car. He wanted to do this so he did not feel so lonely. After the loss of a loved one, I have seen people become very lonely as they spend time grieving. It takes years for them to recover, after having such a loving and fulfilling relationship.

We were driving slowly along the "Spit", near the beach on the Gold Coast, when we noticed a dog sitting still on the front seat of a van, with a seat belt on. It was looking straight ahead and not moving. The owner was camped there on his own, next to the van. The dog caught our attention so we went passed several times and it did not so much as blink. We realised that this dog was dead and had been stuffed. The dog was there to keep the man company. That's how desperate some people become for a loving relationship.

We now sometimes see people with special 'Companion Dogs'. These dogs have permission to be with them where ever they go, they are meant to provide some emotional and relational support and companionship.

Careforce Lifekeys

One of the best programs I have come across that deals with dysfunctional relationships is 'Careforce Lifekeys' It deals with healing wounded and broken relationships. The object is to restore the value of relationships and many other areas of our lives where we may need help. It has been developed by good friends of ours Dr. Allan Meyer and his wife Helen who are based in Melbourne, Australia.

Quoting from one of their brochures they say - *"Lifekey programs can play a key role in enabling people to deal with the issues they struggle with in life by challenging and equipping both wounded and healthy people to live the fullest life possible"*. This covers a wide variety of subjects. I would suggest for further information you contact their website.

Our priority should be our relationship with God

As we enter the twilight years our relationship with God should be our number one priority. In Matthew 22:36-38 we read that a lawyer asked Jesus *"Which is the great commandment in the law"*. Jesus replied, *"You shall love the Lord you God with all your heart, with all your soul, and with all your mind." "This is the first and great commandment."* This should be your number one priority. This relationship is developed through prayer, reading the Word, and listening to the Holy Spirit.

I will admit, that I am not the prayer warrior that I use to be years ago. I would fast and pray sometimes for an extended time. I did a 40-day fast when we were on the mission field in PNG, drinking plenty of fruit juice, with a dash of lemonade to keep up my energy levels. I journaled every day during the fast and could write another book on the things God revealed to me during that time. I hardly ever fast these days, but every morning I try to pray and journal first thing in the morning for a short time.

My relationship with God is more in a continual state of awareness of the Holy Spirit. It is more in keeping in tune with the 'still small voice' of the Holy Spirit, and the consciousness that God is with me, to walk with me and talk with me along the way. I think we all need to find what works for us and pursue it.

Jesus said the second greatest commandment in Matthew 22 is to *"Love your neighbour as yourself."* This may be easier said than done depending on how lovable your neighbour is. But the point is that we try and extend love to everyone and treat them like we would like to be treated. By doing this we may win some to Christ.

Do not close the door

Years ago, when our children were still small and I was preparing my sermon I would close my study door to study and pray. When any of our children came and knocked on the door, I would tell them to go away, because I was too busy to see them. One Day one of them was hurting and needed to talk to me urgently, I was about to tell them to go away, and I felt the Lord say to me *"How many people did I shut the door on, and tell to go away"*. I got convicted and was always available after that time. Apart from the obvious, I think the lesson here is also not to be quick to shut the door on a relationship or give up. We need to foster and value our relationship with God, with people, and especially with family as we enter our twilight years. If we do it, it will make life much more enjoyable.

Improve your relationships by putting this into practice -

*Never deprive someone of hope
it might be all they have.*

*Never waste an opportunity to tell someone
you love them.*

*Success in any job is based on your ability
to deal with people.*

Do not expect life to be fair.

(Author unknown)

Chapter 6

'Aging' from a Woman's Perspective

by Caroline Boyle B.Agr.Sc.

After listening to Terry read some sections of the draft for this book I said to him, *"It seems to major on things from a man's point of view, what about from a woman's perspective?"*

To my surprise, he said, *"Well how about you write a chapter?"* To which I agreed. So here goes!

Mark Twain once wrote, *"Age is an issue of mind over matter. If you don't mind, it doesn't matter."* I like that! But let's get real, if it doesn't matter how come there is such an increase in aging women having cosmetic procedures to try and look younger?

University reunion

We have just returned from a sixty-year reunion of my Melbourne University Agricultural Science Group. It was a shock to see everyone as we had aged so much. Some were immediately recognisable but others took some time to work out. We all seemed so old after sixty years. Most of us had put on weight and everyone had grey hair or a rinse. Unfortunately, quite a few had passed away.

As we reflected and looked at old photos it became obvious that age does not do us any favours. Looking at myself as 'Miss Agricultural Science' I thought what has happened to that tall skinny chick?

They are now talking about a reunion in five years- time, realising that there may not be too many of us left by then. Yes, old age seems to creep up on us so insidiously, and there is no escape.

After university – marriage and family

After University I did teacher training graduating ready to teach Science. With my background in Agricultural Science, I decided to head for the country. I ended up at Horsham High School, in Victoria, thinking that I might meet up with a farmer in the area.

I went to a Nurse's Ball in Horsham and had a dance with this handsome young man named Terry. He escorted me home and we kept dating and were married six months later. We look back and joke about the fact that in a way I still married a farmer, because Terry became a pastor, or a spiritual shepherd, like a sheep farmer.

After graduating from Bible College in Adelaide we went

back to Melbourne where Terry entered the ministry, and I taught at University High School. We built our first-ever house in North Ringwood, Melbourne.

A wife and a mother

You may be thinking that as a wife and mother, I have spent a lot of time just following Terry and that in doing so feel a bit second-rate. I have never felt that way as I believe there is no greater calling than to be a wife and mother. God showed me this very clearly. One day, when I was pregnant with Felicity I was bending over and cleaning the toilet, and I thought to myself *"Is this all there is to being a wife and a mother?"* Immediately God said to me *"Jonah"*. Like Jonah, I realised that I was grumbling about something very important. For me, it was making a lovely home environment and raising children in a Godly home. My attitude turned 180 degrees. I've not looked for anything else, and I do like having clean toilets.

We read in the Bible some very wise family instruction for older women, ***"...the older women likewise, that they be reverent in behaviour, not slanders, not given to much wine, teachers of good things that they admonish the young women to love their husbands, to love their children, to be discreet, chaste, homemakers, good, obedient to their own husbands, that the word of God be not blasphemed."*** – Titus 2:3-5. Regardless of what ministry a woman may claim to have we see here that building a family and a home is still a priority for any woman.

Moving to the mission field

I gave birth in Melbourne to our firstborn Amanda, followed by Felicity and Andrew (Sharon was born in Port Moresby). Terry, after a ministry trip to Papua New Guinea, dropped a bombshell. He said he felt God was calling him to PNG to start a Bible College. I could not believe it. We were so comfortable in our new home, and a great church, and now he is talking about moving to PNG. He said it would only be for a year, but it ended up being six years.

Andrew was only five months old when we left. When the plane landed in Port Moresby, three-year-old Felicity called out in her broken English "Where are the coc-odiles?"

We had an adventurous time in PNG. We loved the people and their simplistic faith. It was exciting, as God was pouring out His Spirit and we saw many wonderful things happening – lives were being changed weekly, as people turned to Christ. We built some wonderful relationships with the people in that nation.

The virtuous wife

While we were in Port Moresby, I led a ladies' bible study on 'The Virtuous Wife'. *"Who can find a virtuous wife? For her worth is far above rubies. The heart of her husband safely trusts her, so he will have no lack of gain."* – Proverbs 31:10-11.

As you look into this passage she appears to be like 'Wonder Woman', she is amazing and sets an almost impossible standard. She is industrious, strong, courageous, super capable, managing the affairs of her household, and supportive of her husband. So the question is asked, *"Who can find such a virtuous wife?"* The implication is that she would be a rare woman, and hard to find.

I do not claim to be that wife, but I felt God spoke to me and challenged me personally concerning verse 23. ***"Her husband is known in the gates when he sits among the elders of the land"***. In other words, his reputation is given a boost by having a virtuous wife who is known by others to be so capable and supportive of him. I felt the Lord say, be careful that you also speak well of your husband. I have endeavoured to make a practice of doing this.

When we came back to Australia it became more noticeable in our Aussie culture how some wives were negatively complaining about their husbands. Australians are not always that complimentary and are sometimes quick to criticise. I was reminded of the virtuous wife study and became determined to try and lead by example. As a result, I believe this had a positive effect on others, including Terry, and our marriage.

Living in Lismore

After we came back to Australia Terry became the senior pastor of Christian Life Centre (now Centre Church) Lismore. I returned to casual teaching and was in great demand in the high schools in the area. We ended up building a house again and settled in well. We loved Lismore as a city and it was a good place to raise our children. The church became a great family church and was also pioneering a Christian School, known as Summerland Christian College. We were thrilled with the church and the way the school began to grow and develop. We ended up staying in Lismore for 21 years.

During this time our children were beginning to leave home to further their education, while we were preparing for retirement.

Of course, all this time we were aging. I found it difficult as the children left home one by one. It was wonderful watching them develop and mature. All of them graduated from University, eventually married, and have given us fourteen lovely grandchildren.

My health

I went through menopause which for me was no big deal. I would get severe headaches regularly with my menstrual cycle, but after menopause, the headaches ceased. Every woman seems to get different symptoms at this time, but I was glad when it was all over. According to our son Andrew, during this time, I became more emotional, and quicker to get upset, which caused more tension in our marriage. I cannot remember being like this myself, but it just shows you how your children pick up these vibes.

I did not sense any form of grief or negative emotions that I would not be able to have any more children. If anything I felt a sense of relief and freedom at the beginning of a new phase of life.

I have also had to deal with thyroid issues, surgery for early-stage breast cancer, treatment for skin cancers, a broken leg, a hip replacement, and cataract removal. (starting to sound like an old crock). All these things have taken their toll on my emotions and caused me to feel frustrated that I have had to deal with them. They remind you of the aging process and make you think "What's going to happen next?"

Our finances

Although Terry has written about our finances, I wanted to share my experiences as well. It was during our working years, that I seemed to take charge of money matters. Before the days of personal computers, I kept track of our banking by keeping a tally of our inputs and outputs. I set up a series of handwritten tables and charts so that we could monitor our investments each month. We knew exactly how much debt we had and how much we were paying off. At one point I even found a mistake the bank had made – not in our favour of course – and when I showed the bank they were amazed at my handwritten tables, charts, and calculations. When we retired Terry started doing some of this on his computer.

Helping with housework

We had not been retired long when my daughter Sharon asked me, *"How is it going being retired?"* I answered, *"Nothing has changed."* *"I still do everything around the house while Terry has more time to relax".* So she went and told him to get in and help as we were both meant to be retired. He now vacuums and has some favourite meals he cooks beautifully, like steak and salmon. He is good at doing the dishes and occasionally helps me in the garden. I love the break this gives me.

Intimacy and sexuality

Terry has also written on this subject in the first chapter of this book with my approval. I would just like to add from a woman's point of view our emotional and physical state has a part to play. These are areas that will affect how we respond to sexual advances. Not that our sex life is over – we still find satisfaction but not so often.

One good thing about retirement is that there are fewer distractions, like children wanting attention, there is more time and privacy, and no worries about getting pregnant.

We often express what we want and need, which can lead to a greater degree of intimacy and connection with one another.

However, as we age our bodies are continually changing and we may have to make some adjustments to aid us to enjoy sex.

Retirement and aging

We eventually retired to the Gold Coast and settled in well to the lifestyle. We found it difficult to find a church home after such a great church family in Lismore. However, the years have rolled by and the aging process has taken its toll as I am not involved in church work anymore, apart from an occasional testimony.

An essay, written by Martha Holstein, who is 65 years of

age (seems young to me) reflects 'On being an old Woman'. She speaks of the physicality of aging and how she wants to be and tries to be both 'ageful and proud'. She reminds us that old age is not a status we choose to become; it is a status we inherit simply by virtue of living, and not dying".

Yes, we need to accept retirement as gracefully as we can even though Terry and I have had numerous health issues over the years. We adore our children and grandchildren and love spending time with them at every opportunity we get. I keep a record in my diary of all their birthdays which we try to remember and acknowledge.

Face up to the aging process

Aging as a woman is not easy, given the pressure we feel to remain beautiful and useful. We all have to face up to the aging process. I'm sure we can all identify with some things that happen to us as we age. Here is a list we have to deal with by Therese J. Borchard.

1. **Confront your changing looks** – We notice wrinkles appearing, smile lines, graying and thinning hair, brown spots on hands and face, loss of muscle tone, hanging skin on arms and neck, and hot flushes. Makeup and hair dye helps a little, but we just have to accept the aging process as gracefully as we can.

2. **Identify your masks** – The things we try and hide that make us look ridiculous. Wearing teenage clothes and trying to look so much younger than we are. Terry loved his late sister Lyn she was tall and attractive but in her 70's she sometimes

dressed like a teenager and he would get embarrassed if he was with her because everyone would stare.

3. **Listen to your inner dialogue** – Just as a mask covers up our insecurities, our internal dialogue exposes them. You are old, fat, ugly, and useless. In our mind, we are sending these emails from ourselves to ourselves because of our negative mindset and internal dialogue.

These are things we have to overcome by accepting the aging process. These confronting comments make us feel that we are not alone as we grapple with this stage of life. But we should still do what we can to present ourselves well and maintain our dignity.

Lessened Reserve Capacity

There is an article in 'Perspectives on Aging' on how the major age-related change in the body is a "Lessened Reserve Capacity". It deals with the fact that all organ systems of the body have a substantial reserve capacity to handle life, and how with aging there is a Lessened Reserve Capacity. This shows up in several ways and I could not agree more. These include -

1. **Slowness** – We all become slower with age. Terry says I never walk fast enough and is often a bit in front of me which is annoying. We are told if we learn to pace ourselves we will perform much better.

2. **Stress** – The body calls on its reserves to deal with high-stress or prolonged-stress situations. The effects of stress

tend to be greater on older adults because of their lessened reserve capacity. Being able to pace ourselves in stressful situations appropriately lessens stress as we age.

3. **Homeostatic Equilibrium** – This has to do with the body's internal functions, such as blood pressure, blood sugar levels, heart rate, gastric and bowel functions, and so on. Because of our lessened reserve capacity as we age, we are more vulnerable to illness, disease, and accidents. Once again pacing ourselves seems to be the key to better health.

I can identify with all these things. The one common denominator is that as we age, we need to slow down and PACE ourselves.

I find driving is harder for me these days. Terry loves driving so I get driven around a lot. But because my reflexes are slower as I age I try and remember to take more opportunities to drive.

As a result, I have come to realise that I need to 'be kind to Caroline'. I love to swim but have cut back on how many laps I do. The distance I walk is less than I use to walk. I have found that I have to purposely pace myself more and more as I age, and not try and do things all at once.

Terry is inclined to want everything done yesterday, but I notice that he is also starting to slow down and pace himself.

Family and friends

Terry has written a great chapter in this book on valuing relationships. I think as I get older I value relationships with family and friends more than ever.

I have three sisters, Rosalie, Jill, and Miriam, whom I feel close to even though we are separated by distance. We are living on the Gold Coast while Rosalie, Jill, and her husband Robert are in Melbourne, and Miriam and her husband Phil are in Canada. I also have a brother Norman and his wife Mary who live in Portsea, Victoria.

Our immediate family, all living in Queensland, love getting together for Christmas (all twenty-four of us). It seems that everyone prefers to come to our place. We have such a lovely home that backs onto 'Salt Water Creek', where some go fishing and everyone can spread out and enjoy themselves.

Even though they all pitch in and bring something, by the end of the day I am usually exhausted, and so is Terry, and we long for some respite after they have all gone home.

Don't get me wrong – we love having everyone and it is one of my greatest joys in my retirement years to just be with family and friends.

I hope this chapter has been enlightening for you as a woman. May it encourage you as you near your retirement, and help you enter your twilight years with greater understanding, wisdom, and joy.

Chapter 7

Coping with change

We live in a world that is continually changing. It can be difficult for us to adapt to some of these changes.

Heraclitus, an ancient Greek philosopher said, *"The only constant in life is change"*. That is so true, especially recently due to the Covid-19 pandemic, which has been stressful to deal with because of all the variable changes.

There are many changes in the workforce with increasing automation and technology. I still get in touch with my son Andrew to help me sort out issues with my computer and my mobile phone.

Adapting to change

We can learn to adapt to change as we get older. Healthy aging means finding new things to enjoy and staying physically and socially active. Getting older does not automatically mean that you will be confined to a walker or a wheelchair. (that may happen). But plenty of older people enjoy vigorous health well into their 60s, 70s 80s, sometimes better than those who are younger. You are probably stronger and more resilient than you realize and can adapt to change better than you think.

I was at a church and talking to a man who is 81 and actively involved in both the 'Alpha' and 'Emmaus Walk' programs in his church and loving it.

Some tips to help you adjust to change –

1. Try something new (experiment)

2. Be thankful for what you can do already

3. Try an exercise routine (even just walking)

4. Be positive (look for the silver lining in life)

5. Pick up a neglected Hobby, or start a new one

6. Maintain good relationships or start new ones

7. Accept certain limitations

Dare to take a risk

We need to realize that although change is not easy sometimes it involves taking a risk. Brene Brown, Ph.D., MSW in her best seller 'Daring Greatly' talks about How the courage to be vulnerable transforms the way we live, love, parent, and lead.

The phrase 'Daring Greatly' is from Theodore Roosevelt's speech 'Citizens in a Republic' also known as 'The Man in the Arena', which I prefer. This is an extract of the passage that made the speech famous. *"It's not the critic who counts: not the man who points out how the strong man stumbles, or where the doer of deeds could have done them better. The credit belongs to the man who is actually in the arena, whose face is marred with dust sweat, and blood; who strives valiantly, who errs and comes short again and again there is no effort without error and without shortcomings who may fail but at least fails by daring greatly."*

Brene Brown goes on to state that there is no shame in stumbling, it is a part of the process. Being vulnerable isn't about succeeding or failing it's about being willing to step into the arena and have a go. It is about the one who dares greatly. This is not so easy as we get older, but I hope you get the point, there is no shame if you fail when you dare greatly.

Use the difficulty

I was listening to an interview with British actor Michael Caine. He was asked how he overcame difficult situations. He said when he was a young actor he was meant to enter a room in a scene. When he went to go inside there was a chair in the way and he stopped. The director said, *"Why did you stop?"* He explained that there was a chair in the way. The director said, *"Use your difficulty"*, *"If it is a comedy, trip over it, if it was a serious drama pick it up and smash it."* He never forgot that advice and throughout his career used it to his advantage.

When I heard him tell this story I thought that surely there is a lesson here for all of us. In difficult times when things change and we are caught off guard if we only could learn to use our difficulty to our advantage.

A changing world

We live in a closely connected world, where things that happen in one part of the world will affect other parts of the world. For example, at the time of writing, the Russian invasion of Ukraine continues. This has affected economies around the world, and especially the whole area of supply and demand. But I would like to focus for a moment on technology.

We read in Daniel 12:4 that in the end times *"Many shall run to and fro, and knowledge shall increase."* That was written over two thousand years ago. People are certainly running (or flying) to and fro, all over the world. And of course, knowledge, science, and technology have all increased at a tremendous rate. From the first fragile aeroplanes to jet travel, putting men on the moon, and plans to send people to Mars by 2040.

It would be hard for me to list all the changes I have seen in my lifetime. I remember before the time of refrigerators, going to the ice factory with my dad to get a big block of ice for our ice chest.

There was the milkman, who came around in a horse and cart, to fill up the cans you left with money at the front door. Then if you were lucky he would let you ride around the block on the cart.

Before the days of washing machines, my mum would wash clothes in a trough with a scrubbing board and then put them through a wringer, before hanging them out to dry.

I remember going down to the shopping centre to watch TV (black and white) through the shop window when they first came to the market. People would take deck chairs and sit on the footpath watching!

Not to mention a host of other things. Probably the advent of computers and mobile phones has had the greatest impact in recent years.

As always companies have to keep up with "change" to survive. They have to restructure and re-organise. Work hours have become more flexible and casual to fit in with these changes.

Artificial intelligence

One of the things we will hear more about in our changing world is artificial intelligence. As we age it is hard to get our head around some of these developments. In its simplest form, it is a field that combines computer science and robust datasets, to enable problem-solving. It also encompasses sub-fields of machine learning and deep learning, which are frequently mentioned in conjunction with artificial intelligence.

It enables computer systems to perform tasks normally requiring human intelligence, such as visual perception, speech recognition, decision-making, and translation between languages. This could become a hacker's dream if it is used by criminals.

I do not pretend to know what 'AI' is all about, but I do like the Grammarly programme I am using to help me with this book. If that is in this category then bring it on. If artificial intelligence is used in the right way it could be a real bonus and very helpful. As we age we need all the help we can get, provided we can understand it all.

Identity Theft

Unfortunately one of the things we have to deal with in our changing world is identity theft. This is when someone steals your personal information, such as your social security card number, bank account number, or credit card details. It may happen in different ways, from sifting through trash bins, accessing corporate databases, using computer technology like discarded computer hard drives, or hacking into computers.

Some time ago our bank informed us that our credit card was being used in Europe to purchase items. About $1200 was used for these transactions. The bank was able to sort it out somehow and retrieved the money or suspended payment. We are not sure how this happened, but we suspect someone local where we made a purchase sold our credit card details to overseas identity thieves. We need to do all we can to protect ourselves.

Spiritual identity theft

If you are a Christian the devil will try and steal your identity in Christ. He does this by undermining your self-image. He will condemn you and make you feel unworthy and unloved by God. He will try and make you doubt if you are a real Christian and if possible make you question your faith and your identity in Christ.

No one, including the devil, or the best hackers in the world can ever steal your identity in Christ. The Bible declares *"Therefore if anyone is in Christ, he is a new creation; old things are passed away; behold all things have become new."* – 2 Corinthians 5:17. In Christ you have a new identity that cannot be stolen. You are loved, chosen, forgiven, a son and a daughter of God, and a citizen of heaven.

The Kingdom of God is absolute... But the Church is relative

God and His kingdom are absolute, they do not change. At the heart of the gospel message Jesus preached was the call to repent for the Kingdom of God is at hand. Jesus proclaimed a Kingdom that does not change and is eternally secure, as an alternative to an ever-changing, insecure, temporal world. God himself does not change. *"For I am the Lord, I do not change."* – Malachi 3:6. Again in the New Testament we see that Jesus does not change. *"Jesus Christ is the same yesterday, today, and forever."* – Hebrews 13:8.

However, the church is relative and is subject to change. With every generation, there seems to be change designed to reach each generation. The gospel message is the same, but the presentation of it, to reach people, is changeable. We see this happening today as a result of the modern world of technology. Communication can be through TV, and live streaming of church meetings, using Computers and Powerpoint presentations – also emails and mobile phones for ways of communicating with people.

Many churches are reaching out to the community in different ways, some through Christian education and Schools. Others through food banks, programs for feeding the poor, and opportunity shops.

When we were leading the church in Lismore we concentrated on Christian education. We were fortunate enough to have a lovely location on some 20 acres on the outskirts of the city. As a Board, we planned and developed the school from a small Primary school with about 50 students to an HSC level High school. A lot of credit should be given to my associate pastor and school principal at the time, Rod Dymock, who was ably assisted by the head of Primary, Cobie van Dommele. We also had a great team of dedicated Christian teachers. Rod was followed by Neil Easter as Principal, with other principals following his retirement.

It has now developed with some magnificent modern facilities. The school has always been under the name of 'Summerland Christian College'. Last I heard, it was running over 600 students. As you can imagine it has had a tremendous impact on the rural community in that area.

Adjust to the times

When it comes to making changes we need the wisdom of

God to help us adjust to change. The Church and Christians can always make wise changes because we should be hearing what the spirit is saying to us and the church. *"He who has an ear, let him hear what the Spirit says to the churches."* – Revelation 2:7. We should be up to date with what is happening today, rather than yesterday. My son Andrew reminds me to do updates on my computer for it to work efficiently. We need to be in tune with the times we live in, and what God is saying to our generation.

We should also be wise enough to discern the times we live in. *"...the sons of Issachar, who had an understanding of the times, to know what Israel. ought to do"* – 1 Chronicles 12:32. This was at a crucial time in history when the Kingdom under Saul was about to be handed over to David. It was time to make David king over all of Israel, and the wise sons of Issachar supported the timing of this change. The people and the tribes were all of one mind to make David King over all of Israel.

A Danger for the church today

Although we need to adapt to change and make adjustments to reach people with the gospel we need to be careful we do not compromise the basic message of Christianity.

William Booth was an English Methodist preacher who founded the Salvation Army. When he was asked what he thought the chief danger of the 20th Century Church would be he answered –

"Religion without the Holy Spirit",

"Christianity without Christ",

"Forgiveness without Repentance",

"Salvation without Regeneration",

"Politics without God".

These words have proven to be prophetic as unfortunately, we see these things happening in some circles of Christianity today.

Change can be uncomfortable

As we get older we seem to feel much more comfortable with regular routines. We do not like changes that make us feel uncomfortable. But sometimes we just have to adjust and step out in faith and embrace changes. I can hear all the people in their twilight years saying very softly *"Amen"*. This also applies of course to Church leaders, and Churches, who have had to make a lot of necessary changes lately largely due to Covid-19 restrictions.

The Lord instructed Abram (Abraham) ***"Get out of your country, from your family, and from your father's house to a land that I will show you."*** – Genesis 12:1. But, he was told if he went he would be blessed, and become a great blessing. In Hebrews 11:8 we are told, ***"He went out not knowing where he was going"***. So he stepped out in faith and obeyed God.

This was a process, as most changes are done step by step. We can learn a few things from this regarding major changes:

- He had a word from God

- He was willing to obey and step out in faith

- He had to leave his roots (his father's house)

- He had to leave his comfort zone

- He was not sure how things would end up

- He believed this move would be blessed.

This no doubt would have been an uncomfortable time in the life of Abram and his family as they stepped out in faith.

Transplanting a Bible College from Melbourne to PNG

When God called us to PNG. I was an assistant pastor to Hal Oxley at Life Ministry Church in Melbourne. It was a thriving Charismatic church.

The church had founded Life Ministry Bible College. It was a great college and I was one of the lecturers together with mainly Hal Oxley, Delton Gordon, Alan Vandenberg, and a host of visiting speakers in those early days of the College.

The calibre of the students was outstanding, many of them ended up in some form of ministry or became influential in their church and community.

As a family, we were very comfortable, we had just built our first home in Melbourne. Then miraculously the call of

God came to go and start a Bible College in Port Moresby. It was like transplanting the college in Melbourne as I used most of their curriculum.

For us, as a family, the transition was a very uncomfortable time. But the College, and our time in PNG, (six years) ended up being a blessing to us and many others. The college impacted the nation.

A continual state of transition

If we look at life from a philosophical point of view we are in a continual state of transition. On the law of averages - from a baby to a teenager to adulthood, from a single person to a married person, raising our children who eventually give us grandchildren, all the time we are aging through to death and then hopefully Heaven. In that time frame, we will, of course, transition from Primary school to High school, and possibly University. Then we are transitioning through our working years with promotions and job changes through to retirement.

From a Christian perspective -

1. God remains the same

2. In Christ, we are changing daily

3. Your current season prepares you for the next.

We have many inspirational bible stories about change and transition -

- Joseph's transition from prisoner to Prime Minister.

- David's transition from shepherd to King.

- Jesus' transition from Heaven to Earth.

- Jesus' transition from the Earth back to Heaven.

- Jesus' disciples transition from working to Apostles.

- Paul's transition from persecutor to Preacher.

Entering into our twilight years, I am not expecting any dramatic changes and challenges, like in my younger years in the workforce or ministry.

One day at a time

We do have a responsibility to cope with changes. Even if it means surviving one day at a time, addressing health issues, paying the bills, fostering relationships with family and friends, and hopefully finding and settling into a church home.

There was a lovely old lady I used to visit when I was pastoring in Lismore who would usually play her favourite song for me which was *"One day at a time sweet Jesus, that's all I'm asking of you, One day at a time."* I will never forget that, and today I often find myself singing it.

If we are to enjoy our twilight years, may God help us to find grace to cope with the challenge of changes, and adapt to them!

Chapter 8

Leaving a legacy for the future

I would like to think that approaching the twilight years we can look back with satisfaction knowing that we have left a legacy that will impact generations to come.

What does it mean to leave a legacy? It means putting a stamp on the future by making a substantial contribution to future generations. We usually want to leave a legacy, because we feel that our life has mattered. If we know what kind of legacy we would like to leave, we should start working toward it.

A legacy is something passed on by or received from an ancestor or predecessor. Leaving a legacy is important for many reasons. It can serve as an example for future generations, preserving memories, and teaching valuable life lessons. It is a source of motivation, inspiring others to aim for greatness despite their circumstances. It is also something for us to strive for regarding leaving a legacy for family, friends, the workplace, and various organisations that we may have been involved in.

The City of Brisbane will host the 2032 Olympic Games, which means the nearby Gold Coast will also be hosting some events. In the 'Gold Coast Bulletin' on Thursday 23 March 2023 there is a heading "Gold Coast Legacy wish list from the Olympics." It is all about what kind of legacy the Olympics will leave the Gold Coast in the future. Things like sporting venues, rail links to the airport, improved road and transport upgrades, and a list of other possible infrastructure as a result of the Olympics in 2032.

Anybody can leave a legacy

We do not have to be famous to leave a legacy. All of us will leave a legacy through the way we live and relate to others. That's what people will remember about us. A book by Merle R. Saferstein 'Living and Leaving My Legacy' shares carefully curated excerpts from over forty years of her journaling. Each is a sample of her life, as she shares the good and bad, the easy and the difficult, the challenges and the breakthroughs. Her journal formatted into a book is an inspiration to many. The point is no matter who you are your life has something to share that can be a legacy that will help others.

We see the desire of King David is clear. He desired to pass on what God had taught him to generations to come. *"O God you have taught me from my youth"*… *"When I am old and grey-headed, Oh God, do not forsake me until I declare your strength to this generation, your power to everyone who is to come."* – Psalm 71:17-18. David put so much value on what God had taught him that he wanted those things passed on from generation to generation. Do you value what you have been taught from the experiences of life? Do you want to pass them on in some way?

A legacy for our children and grandchildren

Legacy focuses on what endures the test of time, and what can be passed on to others who will live on after us. Today we mostly think about passing on a legacy in terms of material things. I remember my parents leaving a list of things that were to be passed on. But leaving a legacy goes much deeper than that. It involves certain principles that we have learned through life, including Godly qualities and eternal values that will impact generations to come.

"A good man leaves an inheritance for his children's, children." – Proverbs 1 3:22. This is primarily talking about money and material possessions. But the same can be said about leaving an inheritance or legacy of values, that we have been able to impart that will in turn be passed on to following generations. We may not leave as many material things as our family hopes to inherit. But I would like to think that I have passed on Christian values to our children that will flow on through their children (our grandchildren) for generations to come.

Our son Andrew is a Baptist minister at the time of writing

and by the grace of God, our children love and follow the Lord. After many years in ministry, nothing thrills me more than to see not only our children and grandchildren living Godly lives but also many others that have thanked me for the input I have had on their lives.

School teachers and Schools

Schools and in particular school teachers can have a tremendous impact on our lives. They may not realise it but they have the potential to influence us greatly. I can still vividly remember teachers back as far as my primary school days.

One teacher that impacted my young life was Miss Devlin. I had her as a teacher in grades two, three, and four. Every 'Remembrance Day' when we had two minutes silence at 11 am she would be at her desk weeping. Her fiancé had been killed in action. She was a lovely lady and a good teacher. One day she cleaned out the draw in her desk and she had us all line up to get something. When my turn came I was given a brown paper bag. When I looked inside it contained bulbs. I was a little disappointed, but I took them home and my mother planted them. They were daffodils and every year when they bloomed, I would think of Miss Devlin. I also remember Mr. Wallace in grade five, and Mr. Parker in grade six with their unique teaching styles. Many High School teachers also had an impact on my life, but none as much as Miss Devlin.

The Christian School, we helped develop during our time in Lismore has had a tremendous impact on the local community. Due to great Christian teachers, I now see former students who have now become parents – some of them have even become teachers in the school and are now sending their children to that school.

The Bible College we establish in Port Moresby PNG years ago has impacted that nation. Many of the students have now become fathers in the faith – quality men and women who are passing on the gospel for generations to come. Others have become businessmen and influential leaders in the community, contributing to the work of the Lord.

Changing someones destiny

I had one senior leader come to me when I was ministering at a leader's conference in Port Moresby recently. He told me that I was ministering in the city of Lae many years ago when he was a young man. He was standing in the foyer of the church listening, but not game enough to come inside. At the end of my message, I had a word of knowledge and said there was a young man in the foyer that needed to come and receive Christ. He said he went home but knew it was him. He could not sleep so he came the next night and stood in the same place. When it came to the altar call, again I said that the same young man who was meant to come forward is standing in the same spot, so please come forward tonight. He did and was saved. He became an influential church leader in his province in PNG.

Legacies are not just those things left behind on earth, but they can go on into eternity because they have been engraved in the lives of those that you have had around you. I am eternally grateful to many people that have had an impact on my life, and I believe the legacy they have passed on to me I have been able to pass on to others.

Thank God for the Bible

The Bible is a legacy that has been left to us by those who took the time to write down and record events as they were inspired by the Holy Spirit.

Consider the impact of the original manuscripts that have been translated into the Bible. *"This will be written for the generation to come. That a people yet to be created may praise the Lord."* – Psalm 102:18. Thank God we have a written legacy in what is now the Bible. The authors were inspired by God to write down things that are now inspiring generation after generation to put their faith and trust in the Lord.

What kind of legacy have people left you? Have they helped you or hurt you? Then ask yourself what kind of legacy will you leave behind. How will people remember you? What will they treasure because of your input into their lives?

Avoid self-centeredness

It is so easy to become self-centered and selfish, especially as we grow older. We can become so consumed with surviving. It is never too late to do some mentoring or to help someone in some way. Isaiah the prophet warned King Hezekiah that the day was coming when all in his house, and his father's house, would be carried away to Babylon, including his entire family and his descendants. Hezekiah's reply to Isaiah was, *"The word of the Lord which you have spoken is good!"* For he said *"Will there not be peace and truth at least in my days."* – 2 Kings 20:16-19.

It is astonishing, firstly, because he says it's a good word. It is far from a good word. Secondly, it is like he is saying *"Who cares, as long as I have peace and truth in my lifetime."* It seems as though he has become so self-centred that he does not care what happens to future generations, as long as all is well with him. Thirdly, you think he would have shown some concern and sought the Lord as to how this could be avoided. He could have at least asked the prophet Isaiah if there was something he could do to save future generations from going into captivity. Of course, we all want peace and truth in our lifetime but that is no excuse for us not to be concerned for future generations.

But surely we want the same and better for our children and grandchildren. Throughout the Bible, we see that God is concerned for the welfare of future generations.

Passing on the baton to others

I remember running in relay races at school and how terrible you felt if you dropped the baton. When I was a teenager I was asked to run in a special Footballer's 400m relay race representing Horsham Football Club at a Stawell Gift meeting. I wanted to start the race, as I thought there was less chance of me dropping the baton. Well, we didn't drop the baton but unfortunately, we came in second place.

Paul in his writings to Timothy refers to the baton of the Christian faith being passed on to others *"The things that you have heard from me among many witnesses, commit these to faithful men who will be able to teach others also."* – 2 Timothy 2:2.

Now, that you are older you might be feeling that you do not have the opportunities to be able to do this today. Perhaps you will still have the opportunity to impart something of value to your family that will last for generations to come.

Paul remembers how the baton of faith was passed on to Timothy through family members. *"I call to remembrance the genuine faith that is in you, which dwelt first in your grandmother Lois, and your mother Eunice"* – 2 Timothy 1:5. We see here that Paul recognizes the importance of previous generations and the impact they can have on us today. The faith he sees in Timothy began with his grandmother and was passed on through his mother, to him.

I'm sure some of you can identify with this. I know I can because my mother had faith in God and said to me one day, *"I would not be surprised if you ended up in the ministry"*. She would not have realised how prophetic that was at the time.

There is no greater joy than to know that you are leaving behind a legacy as you enter the twilight years of your life. If you haven't already, ask God about the legacy He would like you to leave while you still have time.

Chapter 9

How much does God love you?

From a worldly point of view, love is usually thought to be something you receive or give, because you deserve it, or you have earned it.

Like the lyrics to the famous Beatles song -

'Can't buy me, love'

I'll give you all I've got to give

If you say you love me too

I may not have a lot to give

But what I got I'll give to you

I don't care too much for money

Money can't buy me, love

Can't buy me, love

Everybody tells me so

Can't buy me, love

No, No, No, No.

No, Money can't buy love, but the song still implies you have to earn it somehow. The love of God cannot be bought, it is not gained by anything we do. That is why He sent Jesus, to save us from our sins, His love is steadfast and unchanging.

As you enter your twilight years, you may have difficulty understanding how much God loves you. He loves you, not because of who you are or what you've done. God loves you because of who He is. When we doubt God's love for us, it is usually because we have taken our eyes off Him. We start focusing on ourselves, our sins, our insecurities, our shortcomings, and our disappointments.

We may know how much God loves us from a theological point of view but have trouble with it in reality. So we begin to wonder if He does love us. Sometimes we feel forgotten or overlooked because of the circumstances we may be facing, especially if we are grieving the loss of a loved one, struggling with health issues, or battling financially, or if we are in a broken relationship, or experiencing some kind of opposition.

Unconditional love

The love of God is unconditional. No matter what you are going through or how unworthy you may feel at times, His love is not based on your feelings or your performance.

Religion and legalism demand you have to obey all the rules before you are validated by God. The Bible says, *"But God demonstrates His love toward us, in that while we were still sinners, Christ died for us."* – Romans 5:8.

This is unconditional love. We see how God demonstrates His love for us. While we were still sinners He sent Christ to die for us. I have done things I am ashamed of and I am well aware that I do not deserve to be loved by God. I am very aware that I am a sinner saved by grace. I marvel at His love and often sing to myself the old Hymn –

"I stand amazed in the presence of Jesus the Nazarene, And wonder how He could love me a sinner condemned unclean, How marvelous, how wonderful and my song shall ever be; how marvelous how wonderful is my Saviours love for me".

There are no demands or conditions. When it comes to salvation there are no strings attached. He did not say after you repent, study the bible, go to church, or pray I will love you.

It is because of His unconditional love, we all have the opportunity to repent and accept Christ as our Saviour and Lord. We have no excuse for not repenting. His love is unconditional for the whole human race. It is up to us to respond.

Having said all that, all of the above disciplines will help us develop a closer relationship with God, which should make us more aware of His love for us.

God confirming His love for me

I want to tell you an incredible story, it is almost unbelievable. But before I do I want to back it up with a scripture *"He chose us in Him before the foundation of the world, that we should be holy and without blame before Him in love."* – Ephesians 1:4

When I was about 14 years of age (I was not a Christian at the time) I went on a long weekend fishing trip with my father. We camped on the shores of Lake Wartook in the beautiful Grampian Mountain Range, near my hometown of Horsham, Victoria. We arrived on Saturday and launched our little tinny and motored over and dropped anchor near an outlet tower on the lake. Straight away fish started biting furiously. We were catching Redfin or English Perch one after another. I have never seen anything like it, before or since that day. We had garden worms for bait but in the end, all we had to do was drop a bare hook in the water to catch them. We had fish all over the bottom of the boat. Then as suddenly as they started biting they stopped.

We had so many fish and no way of keeping them fresh so we decided to take them home and come back the next day. When we got home we laid them out on the front lawn and invited our neighbours to come and take some. They were good size eating fish from around a pound to three pounds in weight.

Before anyone took some my father said *"Terry count them"*. I counted them very carefully. Guess how many? Exactly 153.

The next day we went back and fished in the same spot and did not even get a bite. The rest of the weekend we caught nothing.

It was years later after I became a Christian that I discovered the scripture where the disciples caught 153 fish. ***"Simon Peter went up and dragged the net to land, full of large fish, 153; although there were so many the net was not broken."*** – John 21:11.

When I read this scripture, the Lord remind me of the 153 fish I caught with my father that day. It was no coincidence. I felt the Lord speak into my heart and say, *"I just wanted to let you know that I loved you and chose you before the foundation of the world to be one of my disciples."* It was as though the Lord was confirming the calling I had on my life to be in the ministry.

Attachment to God and prayer

According to a 'Baylor University Study', *"As people grow older those who are securely attached to God are more likely to have a sense of wellbeing, and the more frequently they pray the greater that feeling"*. *"But those who feel more distant from God do not have the same benefit."*

A study published in the 'Journal of Aging Health' focuses on three measures of health, *"Optimism, Self-Esteem, and Contentment with life, and shows that for all of them, there is a relationship between attachment to God and prayer"*.

Yes, God loves us but we become more aware of it when we are attached to Him and relating to Him in prayer.

God will stand with you

No matter what you might be experiencing, or what doubts you may have about God's love for you, God will stand with you. He will never abandon you.

The Apostle Paul went through a stressful time, where he faced disappointment, opposition, and isolation. I refer to 2 Timothy 4:9-17. *"Demas had forsaken him, having loved this present world. Alexander the coppersmith did him much harm"*.

When Paul tried to defend himself he said *"No one would stand with me, they all forsook me."* Then in verse 17, we read Paul declaring *"But the LORD STOOD WITH ME, and strengthened me"*. I love that, *"But the Lord stood with me"*. Not only did the Lord stand with him but also strengthened him in his time of trouble.

As I look back over my life, I have faced disappointment, opposition, and isolation. But I can also say that *"The Lord stood with me,"* and strengthened me. When I was diagnosed with prostate cancer and had to undergo six weeks of radiation treatment, and read about the possible side effects, I felt like not going ahead with the treatment. But the Lord spoke a word into my heart, *"You will get through this for I am with you"*. It was tough at times, but He stood with me. I was able to endure the treatment with minimal side effects. The result after my treatment and blood test was perfect. My PSA read 0.01 which is as low as you can go, and no sign of cancer. Praise God! Yes, the Lord does love you, and will never stop loving you. He will stand with you no matter what you might be feeling or experiencing.

Like or love?

When I first started preaching on the mission field in PNG, I became frustrated trying to convey the fact that God did love people. I was preaching through an interpreter who was translating my English into Pidgin English. I said that *"God loves you"* and the interpreter said in Pidgin *"God emi laikim yu"*, which in English is *"God likes you"*. I stopped the interpreter and said, *"No I did not say 'like' I said 'love'."* To which the interpreter said I am sorry but there is no word for 'love' in Pidgin, 'like' is the best I can do. I felt that was completely inadequate, imagine me telling my wife I liked her. It's just not the same.

We have all heard people use phrases like *"I love you to the moon and back"*, *"I love you heaps"*, or *"I love you forever and ever"*. These are expressions that try and convey, just how much they do love someone. On the other hand, love can be used casually, like *"I love my job"*, *"I love my house"*, *"I love my car"*, *"I love my city,"* or *"I love sport"*.

When God says He loves us, we usually accept it by faith, because He has revealed His love to us through His forgiveness, His mercy, His grace, and His sacrificial death on the cross, which assures us of eternal life if we believe in Jesus.

Consider the greatest 'adverb' in the Bible

Some scriptures try and convey to us just how much God does love us. Take for example one of the greatest 'adverbs' in the bible. An 'adverb' to me (and I'm no English teacher) is adding more meaning to a 'verb', it gives the verb in a sentence more power. When we read John 3:16 *"God so loved the world"*. 'Loved' is the verb, but 'so' is the adverb.

This gives more meaning and weight to the fact that God really does love us, He loves us 'so' much that it leads to another verb, telling us how and why He loves us. The next verb is 'gave', He 'gave' us His son Jesus Christ, *"That whoever believes in Him, should not perish but have everlasting life."*

This emphasises and empowers the fact that God loves us. He loves you and died for you. If you haven't already received Him as your saviour and Lord, ask Him right now to come into your life and forgive you and save you.

Love through actions

I was leading a home group in Melbourne years ago in our home, and we had the late David Muap from PNG visit one night. It had been raining and everyone left their shoes at the front door. One of the men in the group asked me for some shoe polish, and while we were having supper, he went and polished David's shoes, which were in bad shape. It is these little acts of love that we remember, more than all the sermons we hear on love.

I will never forget a visiting speaker we had from America, ministering for us when we were in PNG. His theme was 'love' and he brought some great messages about love. In one of the night meetings it turned very cold (which was a rare event in

PNG). He saw me shivering in the front row (most unusual) and took his jacket off and gave it to me. After the meeting when I went to give it back, he insisted that I keep it. I valued that jacket, and every time I wore that jacket years later, who and what did I think about? Yes, I thought about that man and the love that he brought, not only through his words but also through his actions.

Making someone feel loved

There was a scene in the movie 'A Beautiful Day in the Neighbourhood' that touched my heart. A journalist was asked to investigate this man who hosted a children's show on TV, Mr. Rogers (played by Tom Hanks), because he seemed too good to be true. The journalist had an appointment to interview him but it was not possible as they ran out of time.

So Mr. Rogers rang the journalist that night to do a phone interview. He begins the conversation with *"Would you like to know what I am doing tonight?"* To which the journalist replies *"Yes, what are you doing?"* Mr. Rogers replies, *"I am doing the most important thing in the world right now".* To which the Journalist replies, *"and what is that?"* Mr Rogers replies *"I am talking to you."* Some people seem to have that ability when you talk to them, to make you feel like you are loved, and the most important person in the world.

Nothing can separate you from His love

We may feel at times that many things separate us from His love. When we go through difficult times we tend to react by thinking God has forsaken us.

However, we read in Romans 8:35-39 *"Who shall separate us from the love of Christ, tribulation, distress, persecution, famine, nakedness, peril, or the sword?" "For I am persuaded that neither death nor life, nor angels, nor principalities, nor powers, nor things present, nor things to come, nor height nor depth, nor any other created thing, shall be able to separate us from the love of God which in Christ Jesus our Lord."* Notice it starts with WHO can separate us from the love of Christ. Some people may be involved. So we need to be mindful that NOBODY and NOTHING can separate us from His love.

Some years ago we were traveling in a very remote desolate area in Western Australia. We were traveling along an extremely rough road when my wife said *"I think we have a flat tire."* I was in denial as I did not want to stop in the heat, in the middle of such an isolated wilderness. But by the time I stopped the tyre was completely shredded. Then suddenly out of nowhere a (so-called) ranger drove up, stopped, and changed the tire for me. Then he told me to go back to the coast to get new tires, as we would not get any heading further inland. We went back about 200 km to the coast. Finally, we got the tires we wanted only because they were on back order that someone had failed to pick up. We are convinced to this day, the ranger was an angel.

That night I was reading from Romans 8 *"NOTHING can separate us from the love of God in Christ Jesus our Lord."* We left very early the next morning and drove some 300 km back inland to a remote mining town. Pulled up in front of a little Baptist church, in time for their Sunday service. We went inside and sat down and the minister got up and said my text for today is from Romans 8 *"NOTHING can separate us from the love of God in Christ Jesus our Lord."* I had to brush the tears from my eyes, realising how much God, through the events we had just been through had demonstrated and confirmed His love to us.

Despite impending hardships, NOTHING is going to separate you from His love, because He loves you so much.

Some strangers may be Angels

I just mentioned in the story above how we were convinced that the ranger who stopped to help us and guide us was possibly an angel. God because of His love can sometimes send His angels to watch over us at times when we need help. *"Do not forget to entertain strangers, for by so doing some have unwittingly entertained angels."* – Hebrews 13:2. Yes, it is possible that when we have strangers help us at strategic times that we may unwittingly have encounters with angels. You can probably think of times when maybe you have had such a visitation.

There was another time when we were in London and we were on a public bus and we were going to see the Tower of London and the Tower Bridge. I wasn't sure where we were meant to get off the bus so I asked the driver, who was Indian, but I had trouble understanding him. Then an elderly lady sitting opposite us said to me, "It is okay I will show you where, and get off with you". So this lady not only got off with us but proceeded to show us around. She pointed out the Tower of London which we said we would do later. She then took us around St. Katharines Dock Marina (which we didn't know existed) it was lovely, then she took us over to take some photos of the Tower Bridge. When we came to a statue of some dolphins she said this is a popular spot to take photos. After I took some photos with Caroline, I said let us get some photos with this lovely lady. We turned around and she was gone. We looked everywhere and could not find her. We were convinced that she must have been an angel. You may be thinking why would God bother to do that? My only answer is, it was just God loving us His children.

God is so loving, you would have to be crazy to do something stupid that would cause you to turn your back on God, and in doing so, step outside of His protective love. May God give you wisdom and grace to either enter into or stay within the bounds of His love.

As you enter your twilight years, might you be mindful that despite your age and circumstances, you can rest in the fact that God loves you 'so' much!

Chapter 10

Being led by the Holy Spirit

This can be a challenge as most people by the time they reach their twilight years have become very independent and set in their ways. Some Christians will also be in this category.

In our infant years, we are led by parents, relatives and friends. We learn not to touch hot things or things that bite and we are told to look both ways before crossing the road. So as we grow up and become more mature, we are led by our common sense, which tells us there are things we should be cautious and fearful about. So to keep safe we are inclined to stick to our comfort zones.

We usually continue to look for good leadership to lead us as the years unfold. If you were in a battle on the battlefield and you were surrounded by the enemy, who would you follow? You would be expected to follow your senior-ranked officer. But what if he did not know what to do and started to say things like *"I don't know how to get out of this, so I think we should surrender"*? However, if a young private spoke up and said *"I know this area and I can lead you out of this battle"*. Who would you want to follow? I know who I would. The one who knows the way. The Holy Spirit is the one who always knows the way through the battles of life, and the one we should listen to and be prepared to follow.

If you are a Christian by the time you get to be in your twilight years, hopefully, you should be being led by the Holy Spirit. From the time a person places their faith in Christ, they are indwelt by the Holy Spirit, who is permanently with them to lead, guide, comfort and help them through life. This may feel risky at times if we are required to step out in faith.

Another Helper

When Jesus told His disciples He was going to leave this earth and return to the Father He said ***"He will give you another Helper that He may abide with you forever - the Spirit of truth, whom the world cannot receive because it neither knows Him; but you know Him, for He dwells with you and will be in you. I will not leave you as orphans; I will come to you."*** – John 14:16-17. We may not have Jesus literally with us but He is still with us to help us through life as we are led by the Holy Spirit.

It is a wonderful experience to be led daily by the Holy Spirit, as sons and daughters of God. ***"As many as are led by the Spirit of God, these are sons of God. For you did*** *not receive the spirit of bondage again to fear, but you received the Spirit of Adoption by whom we cry out, "Abba Father."* – Romans 8:14-16.

Christians have not received a Spirit of fear, to stay in bondage. We have been set free from our old life, to explore the privilege of being led by the Holy Spirit.

The Dovetailing of the Holy Spirit

I have coined the term "dovetailing" concerning the working of the Holy Spirit in our lives. I have not used this term before or heard it being used, but I dare say it has in this context.

I refer to when certain events dovetail and come together through the leading of the Holy Spirit for a particular purpose. The dove is representing the Holy Spirit which causes things to fit together like a carpenter would make a dovetail joint when putting something together.

When Jesus was baptised by John the Baptist the Holy Spirit descended on Him like a dove *"He saw the Spirit of God descending like a dove and alighting upon Him."* – Matthew 3:16.

This was no accident or coincidence that John the Baptist was baptising in the river Jordan the day Jesus came walking toward him. John announces him as *"The Lamb of God who takes away the sin of the world."* – John 1:29. This was declaring that Jesus was the long-awaited Messiah.

When the Holy Spirit descended like a dove upon Jesus,

the voice of the Father was heard saying *"This is My beloved Son, in whom I am well pleased."* – Matthew 3:17. This was not just two cousins putting on a show. It was God confirming that Jesus was the Messiah. These events all dovetailed together at the right time.

We see this dovetailing repeated again and again in the life and ministry of Jesus and the Apostles. We need to realise that if we are being led by the Holy Spirit we will understand that things are not just happening by chance, they are being dovetailed together by the Holy Spirit.

Spirit, soul, and body

We are made up of spirit, soul and body *"May your whole spirit, soul, and body, be preserved blameless at the coming of our Lord Jesus Christ."* – 1 Thessalonians 5:23. Our spirit is our inner man, the soul is the area of our mind, and the body is our fleshly body that we live in.

The body is very obvious to us all but the soul and the spirit are concealed to the natural eye. The soulish realm could be described as the area of the renewing of the mind which is so important. There are plenty of books and sermons on this subject so I want to deal more with the connection of our spirit with the Holy Spirit within the framework of the inner man and outer man.

The still small voice of the Holy Spirit

We could explore many ways by which we can be led by the Holy Spirit, but the one that has been a help and a challenge to me is what I would like to call being led by the "still small voice" of the Holy Spirit.

I do not want you to get the wrong idea. I am not talking about hearing voices in your head where you may need psychiatric help. But hearing the Holy Spirit speaking into your spirit. *"The Spirit Himself bears witness with our spirit that we are children of God."* – Romans 8:16. We see that the Holy Spirit bears witness with our spirit. How does this happen?

When Elijah fled and hid in a cave. The Lord told him to go out and stand at the entrance to the cave. The Lord passed by and there was a great wind, an earthquake and a fire that hit the mountain near where he was standing. We are told that the Lord was not in any of these great manifestations, but in *"a still small voice."* – 1 Kings 19:11-13. I think coming from a Pentecostal background I would rather find God in the great manifestations of His power.

When I was on what ended up a 40-day fast in PNG, near the end of the fast, I had driven up into the mountains near Port Moresby to pray and seek God. I walked around the bush asking God to manifest himself in a spectacular way expecting some great manifestation. All I got was a still small voice inside me that said *"HERE I AM."* I knew it was God speaking into my spirit, that still small voice was confirmation for me, as I had heard it before and had acted on it, and saw God move as a result.

A Miracle

One example of that 'still small voice' comes to mind that resulted in a miracle. A young couple, graduates from the University in Port Moresby, had their first child, a baby girl. They called her Saua. After several months it became clear that something was not right. Her head began to swell on one side. It was noticeable to everyone. She was sent to Australia where they did several scans and found a tumour in her head. They did a biopsy and found it to be malignant and a fast-growing inoperable tumour. They were told she probably only had about nine months to live. We had prayed for her several times, but there was no sign of healing. Then one Sunday morning just before we were to take communion I heard that 'still small voice' saying inside me, "You have to pray for baby Saua and anoint her with oil". I was sitting next to John Pasterkamp who was about to take communion and whispered this in his ear. John acted immediately took the microphone and told the congregation what I had just said to him, you could feel the people lift their faith to another level. John called the parents to come out the front with Saua and we anointed her with oil and prayed for a miracle. Saua was healed from that moment on. The last time I saw her she was about twenty years of age.

The still small voice is the Holy Spirit bearing witness with our spirit in the inner man. It is not always related to healing but often comes as a word of knowledge or word of wisdom which can also relate to guidance and direction. This 'still small voice' usually comes to me in such a gentle and quiet way, that I can easily miss it. As we are about to look into the inner man, we need to first consider the outer man or natural man.

The outer man

The Apostle Paul gives us some encouragement in our twilight years and nails it when he says *"Therefore we do not lose heart, even though the outer man is perishing, yet the inner man is being renewed day by day."* – 2 Corinthians 4:16. As we age, I'm sure we are very aware of the outward man perishing. We have a limited time left on earth in our mortal bodies. We spend a lot of time attending to the outer man and looking after it as best we can.

However, we see shows on TV like 'Botched' where people go to extremes and spend a fortune having 'makeovers' trying to improve their looks through implants and plastic surgery. Many of these have been botched and look terrible and need to be reconstructed to look presentable.

As we age, our old bodies may need all the help they can get to stay fit and healthy and look good. But because our body is slowly perishing we have to gracefully accept our limitations.

The inner man

I would like to expound more about the inner man. As already mentioned in 2 Corinthians 4:16, *"The inward man is being renewed day by day."*

So we see that the inner man is not going to perish it is being renewed daily, and being prepared for eternity. Peter calls the inner man *"The hidden person of the heart."* – Peter 3:4.

Paul explains that he is already operating under what he calls the law of God according to the inner man. *"For I delight in the law of God according to the inner man."* – Romans 7:22

You have a spirit and the spirit dwells in your body. That spirit or inner man or the hidden person of the heart is the real you. I have been present when several Christians have died. When someone dies they initially go limp like a rag doll. You can sense that the real person (or spirit) has gone to be with the Lord. All that is left is the shell of the outer man.

How do we develop the inner man? Just as we feed our outer man with food, we also need to feed our inner man with spiritual food. We can help develop this area through listening to the still small voice of the Holy Spirit, reading and studying the Word, praying in the Spirit, speaking in tongues, and spending time in fellowship with other believers.

A potential problem

We see in the scripture that the natural man is not capable of discerning the things of the Holy Spirit. *"But the natural man (Non-Christian) does not receive the things of the Spirit of God, for they are foolishness to him; nor can he know them because they are spiritually discerned."* – 1 Corinthians 2:14. Maybe this is why Jesus emphasised that a person *"...must be born again of the Spirit."* – John 3:7-8.

So we have a problem, when the natural man, tries to make himself more spiritual, without first being born again. We end up with a religious person with a form of godliness. They may have head knowledge and know their Bible but are not well able to discern the things of the Spirit if they are not born again by the Holy Spirit.

My wife was from a mainline traditional church. We asked her family minister to marry us. When we told him that after we were married we planned to enrol in a Pentecostal Bible College he became very agitated and tried to discourage us from doing so. I'm not sure what his problem was but the word Pentecostal upset him. I have a feeling he may have clashed with some people from that movement.

Having ears to hear

Jesus said *"He who has ears to hear let him hear what the Spirit is saying to the churches."* – Revelation 2:7. He is not referring to our natural ears, He is referring to our spiritual ears, in the sense that we are hearing and discerning things in the Spirit.

This is important for us if we are to be led by the Holy Spirit. This is where I feel we hear the 'still small voice'. I have found for me to operate in the gifts of the Spirit I need to be hearing or seeing what the Spirit is saying in my spirit. Whenever I have had a word of knowledge or a word of wisdom it is usually a word or sentence I hear or see in my spirit. It seems to be in my spirit or inner man (some would say in your mind's eye). It is hard to give a rational explanation, for it is in the realm of the Spirit. I heard one minister who moved a lot in the Spirit, when asked to explain how it worked for him he simply said: *"You just know that you know, that you know that it is God."* But he could not fully explain it.

In Matthew 13:11 Jesus said to His disciples ***"To you, it has been given to know the mystery of the kingdom of God; but to those who are outside, all things come in parables. Seeing they may see and not perceive, hearing they may hear and not understand."*** This refers to those who are not yet born again. However, if you are a born-again Christian you will be able to see and hear things in the Spirit and perceive and understand them.

Exercising our spiritual senses

We are always exercising the use of our five natural senses, hearing, seeing, smelling, tasting and feeling. Why not exercise our spiritual senses? I would like to think that we have all five of these senses also in the realm of the Spirit.

We read in Hebrews 5:14 ***"Those who by reason of use have their senses exercised to discern both good and evil."*** It would appear that we need to exercise and use our spiritual senses that operate mainly through the area of the inner man to discern what is good and what is evil. But I believe it goes a little further where we discern the things of the Holy Spirit in our spirit.

To give you an example, I knew a Christian leader who not only led his church, but a movement. He told me he was being undermined by somebody. He had no idea where it was coming from. His credibility was being questioned. As he was trying to work it out one day, he saw in the Spirit in his inner man a brown snake winding through a harvest field. He immediately knew in the Spirit that it was one of his elders who always wore a brown suit. He was right. When he confronted the man, the man confessed that he was the problem. He resigned and left the church.

Freely given to us

We do not have to earn the right to hear from God or discern His voice in the inner man. We can take advantage of being able to be sensitive to our inner man that is in tune with the things of the Spirit. *"Now we have received, not the spirit of the world, but the Spirit who is from God, that we might know the things that have been FREELY given to us by God."* The Holy Spirit teaches comparing spiritual things with spiritual – 1 Corinthians 2:10-13

Please note the things which are 'FREELY' given to us by God. We do not have to beg for them, do good works, pray and fast, or by doing other spiritual disciplines. Although all these disciplines are important, the point is the things of the spirit are FREELY given to us, we do not earn or deserve them. We will hear and receive these things as we tune in to our connection with our inner man and the things of the Holy Spirit. We all fall into the trap of thinking we have to earn the right to hear from God. But that is not true. The devil is a master at trying to make us think that we are not worthy or capable of hearing from God.

Other ways the Holy Spirit leads us

There are other ways in which we can be led by the Holy Spirit, which are probably covered in detail in other books. I will just list just a few –

1. Through the word of God

2. By the inner witness of the Spirit

3. Favourable circumstances (an open door)

4. An invitation to minister somewhere

5. An inner peace when making a decision

6. The prophetic word over your life

7. Putting out a fleece (to test the waters)

8. Confirmation from other people

We still need a balanced life

A word of caution, as one of our Bible College lectures, told us *"Do not become so heavenly minded, that you become, no earthly good."* In other words, we have this treasure in earthen vessels, and we are dependent upon our natural bodies to fulfil our spiritual calling here on earth.

I heard a well-respected minister say *"It is perfectly spiritual to be natural, and perfectly natural to be spiritual"*. Our natural man (bodies) are also the vessels God has given us for all kinds of activities and fun here on earth. We should make the most of it while we are still fit and healthy. It is up to us to keep in good shape, to do the things that give us great enjoyment and fulfilment in life.

As we enter our twilight years, and our bodies are not so active, may we become more active in the realm of the Spirit, and aware of the 'inner man' being connected to the 'still small voice' of the Holy Spirit! If you can practice doing this I believe it will release your faith and confidence and give you a more enjoyable lifestyle.

Chapter 11

Meditation and self-talk

This appears to be a passive subject, but it is also a very important one. It does not require a lot of physical activity, which suits us as we enter our twilight years. This is something we can all practice and benefit from.

History records that meditation has been around for thousands of years in one form or another.

In a publication on Self-talk and Meditation - A Lesson for Philosophical Practice by Ran Lahav, University of Haifa Israel and Johnson State College Vermont, says *"The Roman Emperor Marcus Aurelius' papers on 'Meditations' is a fascinating text because it not only presents a deep conception about life but also mentions practical ways of applying this conception to everyday life".*

Prominent historians of Philosophy, Pierre Hadot, and

A. A. Lang interpret it as *"A personal notebook of Stoic exercises, or what Pierre Hadot calls spiritual exercises. His primary purpose in writing this text was not to record his thoughts and actions but to influence them."*

Unfortunately, the Roman Emporers' 'Meditations' was very misguided as he was dedicated to the 'gods' and had thousands of Christians killed in the Colosseum for blasphemy.

Eastern meditation

We are familiar with Eastern meditation because of the emergence of the New Age Movement, which seems to embrace some of the Eastern meditation practices. Variants of this form of meditation have been popularised through Western psychologists, self-help books, and fitness and wellness experts. A lot of Eastern meditation is all about emptying the mind, sometimes through chanting mantras, a Sanskrit term, with 'man' meaning mind, and 'tra' meaning release, which is usually a word or a phrase you repeat during meditation, to release your mind to empty it and connect to essential nature. Those who practice it say they get rid of a lot of negative junk on their minds by doing this.

Just a thought or perhaps a warning, I wonder if this form of meditation could become dangerous and leave a person open to deceiving spirits. Jesus indicated that when a spirit finds a house empty (speaking of a person a demon had left) it is inclined to have access to that house again and enter into it (because the house remains empty) with other spirits and the person could be worse off. (Matthew 12:44-45). The scripture implies that a person would be better off by being filled with the Word of God and the Holy Spirit rather than remaining empty.

Christian meditation

Therefore, Eastern meditation is vastly different from Christian meditation. It is through Christian meditation that we can become more positive toward ourselves and the situations we face. This usually involves improving our self-esteem.

When we recognize our value and talk positively to ourselves we are more likely to work through our problems, make better decisions, and achieve our goals. We learn to break off bad habits, like telling ourselves how dumb and stupid we are at times.

The goal of Christian meditation is to fill one's mind mainly with appropriate scriptures to connect with God. Underlying Christian meditation is in pursuit of a loving God who freely offers His wisdom through His word. Christian meditation traces its roots to the most ancient form of meditation, simply thinking over God's words and His promises. Christian meditation is not emptying the mind but is rather calling to mind, thinking over, dwelling on, and applying the knowledge, wisdom, ways, and purposes of God.

In recent years the technique of mindfulness has become synonymous with meditation. For example, Wikipedia defines meditation as – *"A practice in which an individual uses a technique, such as mindfulness, or focusing the mind on a particular object, thought or activity, to train attention and awareness and achieve a mentally clear and emotionally calm and stable state."*

Sitting on the opposite side of Eastern Meditation is Western Meditation, which is merely a form of study, and storing up knowledge, as a student would for an exam.

How and what to meditate on

Christian meditation and self-talk is the ability to minister to oneself, by meditating (or musing) on the Lord, and his word. The word 'musing' is like a cow chewing the cud. *"My heart was hot within me; "While I was musing, the fire burned. Then I spoke with my tongue."* – Psalm 39:3.

I would often use this principle when I was trying to select a message to preach. When I was meditating on what to preach and a fire started to burn in my belly about a certain thought, I would often take that as an indication to preach on that particular subject.

What should we meditate on and how?

1. **On God Himself** – *"When I remember You on my bed, I MEDITATE upon You in the night watches. Because You have been my help, Therefore in the shadow of Your wings I will rejoice."* – Psalm 63:6-7.

2. **On what God has done and can do** – *"I will remember the works of the Lord; Surely I will remember Your wonders of old. I will also*

MEDITATE on all Your work, and TALK of Your deeds. Your way Oh God is in the sanctuary; who is so greater God as our God? You are the God who does wonders." – Psalm 77:11-14.

3. **On what God says in His word** – *"I rise before the dawning of the morning, and cry for help; I hope in your word. My eyes are awake in the night watches that I may MEDITATE on Your word."* – Psalm 119:147-148.

I heard one minister say that Biblical meditation was like his **'Cabin in the Wilderness'**. It was his quiet place, where he could withdraw from his daily routine and just focus upon the Lord and meditate on His word. It was his time of refreshing where he would find renewed strength and energy for his ministry. We are all victims of busyness, and we live in a world that seems to demand more of our time and energy. May we make more time for biblical meditation!

Meditate on God - Not the enemy

When Joshua was called by God, to lead the people of Israel into the 'promised land', and to drive out their enemies from before them, God instructed Joshua to meditate upon His word. *"This book of the law shall not depart from your mouth, but you shall MEDITATE in it day and night, that you may observe to do according to all that is written in it. For then you will make your way prosperous, and then you will have good success."* – Joshua 1:8.

Surely there is a key here for all leaders. Notice how it

says, it shall not depart from your mouth, which I am sure would have involved self-talk, as well as declaring it to others. This would have also stopped Joshua from meditating on the enemy and the opposition he was facing. The lesson for us is not to dwell or meditate on the enemy but on the word of God. It helps not only to meditate but to speak the word, even if it is only to ourselves, and also when others are around.

As I have mentioned, while I was having radiation treatment for prostate cancer every day over six weeks and the side effects began to kick in, I kept meditating on a word that I felt God gave me in the Spirit based on Joshua being prepared to face the enemy in the Promised Land. The word was *"You will get through this for **I AM WITH YOU.**"* I was facing an enemy but I did not meditate on the enemy I meditated and self-talked on that word every day. I not only got through it – I was completely free of cancer by the end of the treatment.

So we see that meditating upon the word of God is associated with a fruitful and prosperous lifestyle. ***"Blessed is the man who walks not in the counsel of the ungodly, nor stands in the path of sinners, nor sits in the seat of the scornful, But his delight is in the law of the Lord, and in His law, he MEDITATES day and night. He shall be like a tree planted by the rivers of water that brings forth its fruit in its season, whose leaf also shall not wither; and whatever he does shall prosper."*** – Psalm 1:1-3.

Meditation in the new testament

There are not so many references to meditation and self-talk in the New Testament, but they are there. I will refer to a couple of obvious ones.

Once again we have a scripture that applies to those in leadership. Paul writes to Timothy and encourages him to meditate on a list of things. *"Let no one despise your youth, be an example to the believers in word, in conduct, in love, in spirit, in faith, in purity. Till I come give attention to reading, to exhortation, to doctrine. Do not neglect the gift that is in you, which was given to you by prophecy with the laying on of hands of the eldership. MEDITATE on these things."* – 1 Timothy 4:12-15. I think Paul is saying do not forget to do these things. It will help you to focus on them, as you meditate on them.

We also have scripture on meditation that applies to all believers *"Whatever things are true, whatever things are noble, whatever things are just, whatever things are pure, whatever things are lovely, whatever things are of good report if there is any virtue and if there is anything praiseworthy – MEDITATE on these things."* – Philippians 4:8. This scripture is encouraging us to have a positive mindset towards Christian values and ethics.

One of the more subtle references to meditation with an emphasis on self-talk is the story of the woman with the issue of blood. "And suddenly, a woman with a flow of blood for twelve years came from behind and touched the hem of His garment. For, she 'SAID TO HERSELF', *"If only I may touch His garment, I shall be made well."* She was meditating and self-talking in faith that Jesus could heal her.

I will never forget the first healing I received as a new Christian. I had been suffering at times from painful sinus congestion. It was really bad, and I had been reading in James about calling for the elders of the church where it says, let them anoint the sick with oil, and they shall be healed. So I started meditating on this and saying to myself, I am going to do this, and I will be healed. So the next meeting I attended I asked the elders to pray for me, believing I would be healed. When they prayed and anointed me with oil I felt immediate relief and was able to breathe freely without the congestion. About a week later the symptoms came back again and I battled for about a month confessing my healing. It then cleared and has not been a problem since that time. There is no greater joy than for a new Christian to receive an answer to prayer.

We also have other scriptures that could imply some meditation and self-talk. *"Be filled with the Spirit, speaking to one another in psalms and hymns and spiritual songs, singing and making melody in your heart to the Lord."* – Ephesians 5:18-1.

Not vain repetition

However, a word of caution. We are not talking about vain repetition. *"When you pray do not use vain repetitions as the heathen do. For they think they will be heard for their many words."* – Matthew 6:7. Meditation is not to be used as a formula to think that if we keep repeating something, this is how we can twist God's arm to get it.

We meditate on the word so that it is quickened to us by the Holy Spirit who releases faith in our hearts to believe in, and trust God.

In our twilight years, we have plenty of time to meditate and self-talk. We have seen how beneficial it can be for us, and how it has the potential to help us to be blessed and enjoy life more.

Chapter 12

Another wilderness season

By the time you reach your twilight years, you have probably been through several wilderness seasons. The thought of facing another one is rather daunting and you will be wondering how and if you could survive another time in the wilderness.

In our Western world, we like to avoid being uncomfortable in life, because we think we have every legitimate reason for doing so. When we hit the wilderness we usually feel weary and burnt out, and everything seems out of focus, as though we are looking at a mirage and trying to work it all out.

We will all go through many wilderness seasons in our lifetime. A natural wilderness is usually an isolated wasteland, where there is little or no water. It is usually a dry and barren place that is not suitable for long-term living. A spiritual wilderness is a similar place where we go through dry times spiritually. They can be tough times, where we feel isolated and cut off – times where we feel we are not hearing from God and our faith is being tested.

Wilderness experiences remind me of John Bunyan's 'Pilgrim's Progress' which tells the story of Christian and his journey from the City of Destruction (representing a sinful earth) to the Celestial City (representing a glorious heaven). Along the way, Christian encounters dangers, trials, temptations, and disappointments, which are typical of what we can go through in life, especially in our wilderness times.

Just for a little while

The apostle Peter explains these seasons as just for a little while, which I find very comforting. *"For a little while, if need be, you have been grieved by various trials, that the genuineness of your faith, being much more precious than gold that perishes, though it is tested by fire, may be found to the praise, honour, and glory at the revelation of Jesus Christ."* – 1 Peter 1:6-7. These seasons are tough times when our faith is on trial and being tested.

I worked in Kalgoorlie, a gold mining area in Western Australia, for a while when I was younger. I would visit the gold mines and watch them pour the gold. During this process, the dross on top was skimmed away until it was pure gold. It would seem that God is doing a similar thing with us in the wilderness.

A time of preparation

It is interesting to note that Jesus was led by the Spirit into the wilderness. *"Then Jesus was led up by the Spirit into the wilderness to be tempted by the devil."* – Matthew 4:1. He was being prepared for His ministry by having to overcome the temptations of the devil. After He fasted forty days and nights he had His encounter with the devil. He resisted and overcame all the devil tempted Him to do, by saying *"It is written"* quoting appropriate scriptures each time.

After Jesus overcame the temptations, we are told *"Now when the devil had ended every temptation, he departed from him until an opportune time."* This would imply that the devil would be back again when he felt he had an opportunity. It is the same for us after having a victory we can not afford to let our guard down because we know he will seek another opportunity to have a go at us.

"Then Jesus returned in the power of the Spirit." – Luke 4:13-14. Yes, Jesus was being prepared and empowered in the wilderness. I would like to think that we are somehow more empowered by the Holy Spirit when we go through a wilderness season.

Sin lies at the door

The devil often tempts us when we are most vulnerable. He wants us to fall into sin to try and destroy our life and ministry. I have seen and heard of several well-known ministers over the years succumbing to temptation and as a result ruining their ministry, marriage, family life, and friendships.

"Sin lies at the door. And its desire is for you, but you should rule over it." – Genesis 4:7.

Sin is never far away, it is like a predator waiting to ambush us. We need to be aware of our weaknesses which often show up when we are in the wilderness. We are meant to be on guard, resist temptation, and rule over it.

I was on a ministry trip in Thailand traveling with Denis Barnard and the taxi driver kept saying to us in his poor English *"A message"*. We thought he had a message for us. Then he showed us some photos and we got the message, he was saying *"massage"*. He was trying to take us to a 'massage parlour'. So we quickly said, *"No, we were happily married"*.

Learn to resist the devil

I have taught a lot about spiritual warfare over the years. As we enter our twilight years we are inclined to slacken off in this area. We just can't be bothered with the devil. However, he will still give us a hard time if he can.

I believe the key word for us as we age and encounter the attacks of the devil is the word 'resist'. It means to stand against and oppose by continual resistance. The inference is that if we will do this he will eventually back off. Paul, Peter, and James all use the word resist when referring to overcoming the devil. *"Therefore submit to God. Resist the devil and he will flee from you"* – James 4:7. This is exactly what Jesus did. He entered into a war of words by quoting scriptures to resist and overcome temptation

I would encourage you to do the same when you feel you are under attack or being buffeted by the devil in some way. Make a stand, and resist until you break through into victory.

Job refused to believe he was being punished

Some people feel they are being punished when they go through a wilderness experience. No, God is not punishing us He is preparing us by testing our faith in difficult situations.

Job did not think he was being punished, despite his suffering, lack of support, criticism from others and not being able to hear from God. He knew he was being tested for some reason. *"Look I go forward, but He is not there, and backward, but I cannot perceive Him"* … *"When He has tested me I shall come forth as gold."* – Job:23:8-10.

His friends and his wife were not much help. His wife said to him, *"Do you still hold fast to your integrity? Curse God and die!"* – Job 2:9. Job gave a wise answer to his wife, he said, *"You speak 'as' one of the foolish women"* – Job 2:10. He did not say she was foolish. He said 'as' one of the foolish women (a lesson for all husbands). We also need to remember she would have been grieving having just lost 10 children.

Some of his friends were suggesting to him that he must have sinned against God, and was being punished for it. Some of our friends may wonder what we have done to be going through a wilderness experience.

Similarly, when Jesus encountered a man born blind the

disciples wondered who had sinned – was it his parents? The prevailing view in the culture was that hardship, calamity, and misfortune must somehow be linked to previous wrongdoing. Many people today, (including some Christians) hold similar views like 'what goes around, comes around' or 'that's just karma.' But Jesus explained to his disciples that no one, including the man himself, had sinned, and that in this case, the man's blindness would eventually bring glory to God when he was healed by Jesus.

Fear and depression may lead to a death wish

Some people when they go through a severe wilderness experience become so fearful and depressed, they wish they could die. Elijah when he was on the run fleeing for his life, *"He went a day's journey into the wilderness, and came and sat down under a broom tree, and he prayed he might die, and said "It is enough! Now Lord take my life."* – 1 Kings 19:4. Elijah did not recognize that God would use this wilderness experience to prepare him for his future.

This also raises another issue for those who are suffering and want to die. 'Voluntary Euthanasia'.

From a Christian perspective if you are sick, suffering, near death, and ready for Heaven, why not consider Voluntary Euthanasia?

I'm referring to 'Active' euthanasia which is killing a patient by active means, for example, injecting a patient with a lethal dose of a drug. It is a controversial issue as some governments have accepted it, and others are trying to legalise the practice.

Those that are for it argue that an individual has the right to life, then he or she has the right to give up that right. They say that a compassionate society would acknowledge and respect that right.

I am not suffering, in terrible pain, near death, and wishing to die. So I do not intend to judge those who are in that position.

However, theologically, the Bible does not support 'Assisted Suicide'. There seems to be no circumstance that would justify the taking of a life.

Life comes from God and belongs to God. He has numbered our days and we are in His hands when it comes to our time of death. *"Man who is born of woman"…. "his days are determined, the number of his months is with you; you have appointed his limits so that he cannot pass."* – Job 14:1-5. We are meant to do everything we can to protect and preserve life by every means possible. Medical science and technology have been doing all they can in this area.

Sometimes God takes us through suffering to prepare us for eternity. *"May the God of all grace who called us to His eternal glory by Christ Jesus, after you have suffered a while, perfect, establish, strengthen, and establish you."* – 1 Peter 5:10.

As Christians, we are never without hope. It is possible

through faith and prayer for God to heal us. *"Is anyone suffering? Let him pray... "Is anyone sick?" "Let him call for the elders of the church, and let them pray over him, anointing him with oil in the name of the Lord. And the prayer of faith will save the sick and the Lord will raise him up."* – James 5:14.

Discerning the source

A wilderness experience may be the result of several factors. It will help us if we can discern the source. I would like to put forward three suggestions that will give you insight into the conflict that you may be facing in the wilderness, and help you to exercise appropriate faith for victory.

1. **A God-inflicted wilderness**
   This is when God is in this season and wants to get our attention for some reason.

2. **A self-inflicted wilderness**
   This is when we have grieved, resisted, or disobeyed the Holy Spirit in some way. This is often self-inflicted by our unwise decisions and mistakes.

3. **An enemy-inflicted wilderness**
   This is when the enemy has buffeted us. (like Paul's thorn in the flesh). Or when we have encountered the enemy's opposition

The one we have been focusing on is the God-inflicted wilderness. A season where God wants to get our attention for some reason.

A burning bush experience

The wilderness is also a place for 'burning bush' experiences. This is where God gets our attention and speaks into our lives usually for a particular purpose. Just like He did with Moses who had fled to the wilderness. When Moses saw a bush burning on the side of a mountain he said, *"I will go over and see this strange sight why the bush does not burn up"*. When the Lord saw that he had gone over to look. God called him from within the bush *"Moses, Moses"*, and Moses said, *"Here I am."* – Exodus 3:3-4. Then God spoke and gave Moses directions for him to lead the people of Israel.

As a young man, I had left a good job working on the local newspaper in Horsham, Victoria, and went on a so-called working holiday around Australia with two of my mates at the time, Gary and George.

When I eventually returned to Horsham a year or so later the area was in a severe drought. There was no work available except a drought relief scheme with the State Rivers. It was an interesting job where we patrolled the water supply channels from the Grampian Mountains to Horsham. Working on the crew was a father and son team that I was drawn to just like Moses was drawn to the burning bush. They would read their bibles during lunch breaks and out of curiosity I started asking them questions. They had come to start a Pentecostal Church in town and invited me along. I ended up going and this eventually led to my salvation and changed the purpose of my life forever. I call this my first-ever burning bush experience.

God coincidences

God coincidences often happen in the wilderness. When God suddenly does something out of the blue and we say, *"What a coincidence!"* But then we realise that only God could create such an event. We have had many over the years. But we had one recently we were on holiday courtesy of Jill and Robert (my wife's sister and brother-in-law). We were staying at their beach house on the Mornington Peninsula near Melbourne.

My wife Caroline had been in the wilderness in her relationship with her brother Norman for many years, they had not spoken or had any contact for some time. He lived in Portsea, Victoria, and we were living on the Gold Coast, Queensland. However, while we were nearby Caroline thought it would be good to make contact and be reconciled in some way. We tried to make contact with him but failed. Then one day I wanted to buy a new shirt. Caroline suggested I go to a shopping centre in Mornington. Then at the last minute, she decided to come with me. As we went into the entrance to the shops out walked her brother Norman and his wife Mary. We were all startled to see one another and ended up having a very warm and cordial chat. They had been to get something sorted out for their phone but were told they would have to make an appointment and come back later. They did not get what they wanted and I did not find the shirt I was looking for, so you would have to say this was indeed a God Coincidence.

A promise, a process, a promise fulfilled

After I was saved, I believe God had given me a PROMISE, that one day I would end up in the ministry. Then came the PROCESS with my wife and I going to Bible College in Adelaide for two years. When we graduated I thought I was ready for ministry. We then moved to Melbourne. But nothing opened up and I worked in a secular job for a couple of years – it was a wilderness time.

Then the senior pastor called me into his office one day and said, *"I believe you want to be a pastor."* Then he gave me seven names on a piece of paper and said, *"These are contacts our youth made, on an 'outreach' to Healesville. See if you can follow them up and start a church."* Well, we did, but it was a tough time. We had a handful of people come to a public hall for meetings. Then one morning a family of seven turned up, followed by a few more families. After about twelve months, and many hard battles, we had up to forty people in our meetings.

The PROMISE FULFILLED was when the senior pastor asked me to hand the Healesville church over to another talented young man, Hank Oldenhof, and then come and join the ministry team in Melbourne, which was a thriving Charismatic Church. This was the beginning of my full-time ministry.

Part of the package

There is one passage of scripture we probably wish was not in the bible. It is for all Christians and is found in Acts 14:21-23. ***"We must through many tribulations enter the Kingdom of God."***

Nobody likes the sound of many tribulations – which could indicate another wilderness. As Christians, like it or not, wilderness experiences are a part of the package.

Just to finish on a more positive note, Jesus said in John 16:33, *"These things I have spoken to you, that in Me you may have PEACE"*. *"In the world, you will have tribulation"*. *"CHEER UP For I have overcome the world."*

No matter what kind of wilderness you may find yourself in or what the devil throws at you, as you enter your twilight years, you can still have a sense of inner peace and joy, knowing that in Jesus Christ you have the victory.

Chapter 13

An uncertain future

As we enter the twilight years the future becomes very uncertain. As we age, every day is a bonus.

Uncertainty is all around us today. We are concerned about global pandemics, the threat of nuclear war, the economy, and our financial state. Not to mention our health, some of our relationships, and other negative possibilities that may lay ahead. We want to feel safe and would like to think that we are in control of our destiny. The fear of uncertainty is very real and can affect our health and well-being.

We can become anxious about what the future may hold, running through various worst-case scenarios in our mind and worrying about them, rather than focusing on the best possibilities. An uncertain future usually implies a future that is likely to be worse than the present.

Speaking of worst-case scenarios the other day, I dropped my wife off for a swim in our complex. I went down to a waterfront location to eat my Macca's breakfast. When I went to start the car I had a flat battery. To make things worse I had forgotten my mobile phone, but I was able to borrow one from John, a regular walker in that area, who was passing by. I rang 'roadside assist', who confirmed that they would be there in an hour. I knew my wife would be waiting for me to pick her up. But she does not have a mobile phone. Anyway, she ended up walking back home and then started to think of all the worst-case scenarios. Her immediate thought process was 'has he been in a car accident?' 'Will the police come and say he has been killed?' When I eventually turned up, I think she had mixed feelings, but assures me that she was glad to see me.

Chronophobia

E. M. Cioran in his book 'The Fall into Time' perfectly summarises all that a Chronophobic individual goes through. *"Chronophobia is defined as the persistent and often irrational fear of the future or the fear of passing time. Since time can be considered as a 'specific object', Chronophobia falls under the category of specific phobias. The word chronophobia is derived from the Greek Chronos meaning time, and Phobos meaning fear"*.

The causes of future phobia will vary greatly from person to person. Most experts believe that a highly stressful or dramatic event can suddenly bring on a phobia. For example, if I were to have a serious life-threatening event while writing this book I could experience Chonophobia by fearing I would run out of time and die before I finished the book, (God forbid).

You can probably imagine similar situations affecting us as we age and realise our days are numbered, and that we may have little time left.

Mind games

Our mind is a minefield that likes to play dangerous games that seem to highlight our fears about all the negative possibilities we may face in the future.

Anisha Petal-Dunn, D.O. says *"Our mind likes to plan for the future using our knowledge of past experiences to anticipate what our future may hold."*

She goes on to say, *"Fear of the unknown causes our mind to worry about the anticipation of the future threat"*. *"Fear of the unknown can trigger the physiological state of stress, which often activates fight-or-flight responses resulting in physical changes, like hormone surges and increased heart rate"*. *"Over time, chronic stress can have a negative impact upon our health, increasing the risk of cardiovascular disease and memory loss."*

Melinda Massoff, Ph.D., a Psychologist, says *"The uncertainty that we are worrying about has to do with our safety and the safety of our loved ones."*

I was playing golf with a younger man who had recently married. When I asked him if they had any children yet, he said no, we are holding off until world events settle down.

He was referring to several things, but mainly to the Russian invasion of Ukraine, and the fear of a nuclear war.

I have spoken to many other people recently, who have expressed their fears about world events and the uncertain future we may face. Most people seem to find it difficult to plan for the future, with mortgage rates at an all-time high, as well as rents going through the roof. Many have put things on hold for a while.

An epidemic of fear

Jesus implies that fear will be epidemic in the world in these last days, before His return. Fear of terrible expectations. We read in Luke 21:25-28 *"On earth distress of nations, with perplexity, the sea and the waves roaring; men's hearts failing them from fear and the expectation of those things which are coming on the earth, for the powers of the heavens will be shaken."* Jesus' words ring true today, with many fearful of the things happening in our world, and what could take place in the future.

The Bible gives us a list of things that will happen on earth before the return of Christ. We just read there will be 'distress of nations'. Whatever happens in one part of the world, affects other parts of the world. We are seeing some nations struggling with their economies, wars, and rumours of wars. There are outbreaks of sicknesses, diseases, and plagues causing large numbers of deaths (like Covid-19, and its variants). We also see unpredictable weather events increasing, and food and supply shortages, just to mention a few.

Refuse to live in fear

There are plenty of things we could be afraid of in these last days, but if we cave into our fears, it is likely to harm our health and lifestyle. *"Fear involves torment"* – 1 John 4:18.

As we age we are more inclined to be afraid of losing our health, our wealth, and our loved ones. If we allow fear to dominate our lives it is likely to torment us and rob us of our joy.

Fear can release harmful chemicals into the body and threaten our physical well-being. We can feel deflated and defeated and withdraw and in danger of losing our confidence and our faith. We need to refuse to be afraid.

Tormenting fear is not from God. *"For God has not given us a spirit of fear, but of power and of love and of a sound mind"* – 2 Timothy 1:7.

If fear is tormenting you it is not from God. It is a spirit so refuse to entertain it. Rebuke and resist it. Never give in to it. Have faith in God.

A healthy fear of God

There is only one acceptable fear though that we all need. It is a healthy fear of God. A healthy fear of God is more like being in awe of Him. It is a reverence and a respect for Him as God Almighty. This is nothing like a tormenting fear. If you were to ask me what is missing in the world and even in the church today I would say it is *'a healthy fear of God'*.

I'm not talking about being scared of God like Adam

and Eve were after they had disobeyed God. They hid from God because of their sin. Yes, they had something to hide! But, by way of contrast, a healthy fear of God is to have a desire to relate to God because of who He is. If you feel you have something to hide from God and you understand how much He loves you, then you will want to repent and seek His forgiveness. The only thing you will be scared of is not being able to be in His presence.

When I came to Christ I had a fear that I would miss out on being in His presence and with Him in Heaven. I was not scared of Him. My fear was an awe of Him and I wanted to repent of my sin, be forgiven, and be in fellowship with Him. I was scared of the alternative which was to be isolated from Him and be eternally lost in Hell.

"The fear of the Lord is the beginning of wisdom" – Proverbs 9:10. A certain fear of things will give me the wisdom to avoid disaster. I'm not going to jump off a cliff because I know what will happen. A healthy fear of God will give you the wisdom to put things right with God.

Lucifer (Satan) had no fear of God and rebelled with a third of the angels and as a result, they lost their place in Heaven. Do not lose your place in Heaven because you do not have a healthy fear of God.

Yes, I know we are saved by grace through faith in Christ. I love the message of grace. I do not want to diminish grace, but on the other hand, let us not allow grace to diminish a healthy fear of God, which reveals how good God is in sending Jesus to die for us so that we might be saved. This goodness can lead people to repentance, where they can embrace the grace of God for salvation.

Anticipatory anxiety or 'What if'

What is anticipatory anxiety? It is another aspect of a fear of the future. It's excessive worry about potential future events. It can also reflect on what you should have done to change things you were anticipating. But usually has to do with future possibilities and scenarios you are anticipating.

People with anticipatory anxiety often experience panic attacks. The best way to define anticipatory anxiety is that it is the anxiety of 'What If'. I'm sure we all have a dose of this from time to time where we focus on the 'What If' anxiety syndrome.

How should we react as Christians? Should we be going into hiding, stockpiling food, and arming ourselves with weapons? I know of some groups including some churches who have done all of these things out of anticipatory anxiety or a fear of what might happen in the future.

You need to accept a degree of uncertainty as there will always be things that will be out of your control.

'Fear Not' little flock

I have not counted the 'fear nots' in the bible myself, but I have heard others say that there are 365, one for each day of the year. Jesus said in Luke 12:32 *"Do not fear, little flock, for it is your Father's good pleasure to give you the Kingdom."*

As Christians, we feel like a little flock in the world. We feel insignificant, and very much in the minority, and wonder if we can have an impact on the world. But it has given God great pleasure to give us the Kingdom. The Kingdom of God is the only place where people can feel secure in this world today. This is at the heart of the gospel message. Despite the negative possibilities we face in the world today, our hope for the future is in Christ Jesus, our Lord, and Saviour. The Bible says those who do not know Christ are like those who have no hope.

We have been called to go into the world and preach the gospel. Jesus said in Matthew 24:14 "This gospel of the Kingdom will be preached in all the world as a witness to all nations, and then the end will come." So no matter how insignificant, or small, we may feel, God has entrusted to us this great task, of taking the gospel into all the world.

Jesus told us to *"Seek first the Kingdom of God"* – Matthew 6:33. Preaching the gospel of the Kingdom should be the number one priority for the church. It is not a time to withdraw and go into hiding, it is a time to step out in faith, with a message of hope for the world.

Stepping out in faith

Without faith, it is impossible to please God. Even in our twilight years, we need to keep witnessing and sharing the gospel. I feel we need to begin by sowing seeds into people's lives. If you do not see an immediate response, someone else probably will, because of the seed you have sown. I have led many people to Christ because someone else took the time to sow the seed of the gospel in their lives.

Jesus gave us the parable of the sower, sowing the seed of the word (Matthew 13). Our responsibility is to keep sowing seeds in faith. According to the parable, some seeds will fail, but others will fall on good ground and produce a harvest. May we keep sowing and praying for a harvest of souls!

What does the gospel offer today?

1. **An Alternative to a failing world**
   From the time of the tower of Babel, until now, the world has tried to build a utopia. Humanity has failed throughout history to do this. Today we have a very unstable world. The Kingdom of God is the only answer to a utopia.

2. **The only source of hope for a failing world**
   Without Christ, we have no hope for a better future. It is through the blood of Christ that we have forgiveness, salvation, and eternal life. Without Christ, we are still dead in our sins. But now, we are filled with hope for the future.

3. **A place of real peace in a failing world**
   Jesus said, *"See that you are not troubled." Why? "Peace I leave with you, My peace I give to you, not as the world gives do I give to you, let not your heart be troubled, or let it be afraid"* – John

14:7.

There is no need for us to fear the future, if we are in Christ. The world cannot replace Christ with Atheism, Communism, alternative philosophies, or religions. Christ is the only hope the world has for a secure future. There is an Anti-Christ spirit in the world today that according to the bible will become more intense and obvious in these last days

A positive mindset

We need to sometimes get our eyes off all the negative stuff that is happening in our world and focus on things above and beyond. *"Seek those things which are above, where Christ is, sitting at the right hand of God". "Set your mind on things above, not on things on earth"* – Colossians 3:2.

It is a good exercise to think and imagine coming into the throne room of God and acknowledging that He has everything under control and allowing His peace to flood your thinking.

Jesus said to his disciples in John 4:35, *"Behold I say to you, 'lift up' your eyes and look at the fields, for they are already white for harvest"*. Yes, there is to be a great harvest of souls before the Lord returns. As Christians, we can rejoice, have faith in God, and *'look up'* and expect great things.

We have the promise of an outpouring of the Holy Spirit in the last days *"And it shall come to pass in the last days, says God, that I will pour out my Spirit upon all flesh"* – Acts 2:17.

Even though we may be entering our twilight years we can still *'look up'*, *'lift up our heads'*, rejoice, pray, witness, and become involved in the harvest.

Chapter 14

How you can find eternal life

When we enter our twilight years we realize that our time on earth is limited. How long do we have left?

No one knows except God. He knows the exact number of years, days, hours, and seconds we have left on this planet. *"All the days ordained for me were written in your book before one of them came to be"* – Psalm 139:16. We are told if all goes well we can expect a life span of around the 70 to 80 mark or longer. (Psalm 90:10). But it then goes on to say *"Teach us to number our days that we may gain a heart of wisdom"* – Psalm 90:12. Yes, our days are numbered and we should apply them wisely.

Death and taxes

One of the leading figures of early American history Benjamin

Franklin said, *"Our constitution is now established, everything seems to promise it will be durable; but, in this world, nothing is certain except death and taxes".*

We still say the same today. Death and taxes are a certainty. This being true, we should be thinking more about preparing for eternity. I do anyway. After all, we are only a heartbeat away from eternity. What about you? Do you think you have found eternal life?

The quest for eternal life

The quest for eternal life has gone on for centuries. The very earliest written histories reveal that humanity has had the universal desire to live forever, and has sought countless ways to defeat the utterly inevitable date with death. The ancient quest for eternal life was sought through artifacts, divine foods, magical formulas, and elixirs.

Wikipedia in an article on our quest for eternal life states that, 'Eternal life refers to continued life after death as outlined in Christian eschatology.' 'The Apostles' Creed testifies 'I believe….the resurrection of the body and life everlasting'.

In the book of Genesis Adam and Eve were put on probation. If they obeyed God they could live eternally from the Tree of Life. If they disobeyed they would lose that privilege. They disobeyed and lost it. However, in the New Testament, we read that Jesus appears as the last Adam and because of His perfect obedience, He restores to us the gift of eternal life for all believers. (Romans 5:17-19).

Jesus implied that finding eternal life was the greatest treasure you could ever hope to find. Better than silver or gold, better than winning the lottery, better than the best pearl ever found. He said *"The Kingdom of Heaven (or finding eternal life) is like a merchant seeking beautiful pearls, who when he has found one pearl of great price, went and sold all he had and bought it"* – Matthew 13:45-46. This explains how precious it is to stumble across eternal life.

It is worth everything you have. But the good news is that it will cost you nothing, it is free, by the grace of God. All you have to do is believe in Christ, repent of your sins, and acknowledge Him as your Saviour and Lord.

No one wants to die

None of us want to die, but the thought of eternal life has always been appealing. I had one of my grandsons ask me how old I was when I told him, he said, *"Are you going to die soon?"* I said, *"I hope not, but I will die well before you."*

He began to get tears in his eyes, and said, *"But I don't want to die."* He wasn't too worried about me dying, he was more concerned about the thought of dying himself.

The Anzac 'Ode'

On Anzac Day the 'Ode' is always quoted *"They shall grow not old, as we that are left grow old; Age shall not weary them, nor the years condemn".* The thought behind this great quote is that although the fallen in battle have forfeited their longevity and have died prematurely, the consolation is that they will never experience the rigors of growing old.

I heard a song on the radio that grabbed my attention the other day. It was 'forever young' by Alphaville. The Lyrics were –

"Forever young, I want to be forever young,

Do you really want to live forever?

Forever and forever, forever young".

It wasn't so much about eternal life, in fact, in another verse, the words were, *"I do not want to grow old"*. It was all about wanting to stay young forever.

A lovely thought, but unfortunately it is just not going to happen. I would like to think that we will not be old in heaven, but like in our prime, young in appearance.

The fountain of eternal life

I remember being fascinated by a movie when I was a boy where they had discovered the secret to eternal life. In the movie, they discovered the fountain of life, and as long as they kept drinking from this fountain they remained young and would never die.

The only water today that can give eternal life is the water that Jesus offers. Jesus promised the woman at the well eternal life. *"Whoever drinks of this water will thirst again, but whoever drinks of the water that I shall give him, will never thirst. But the water that I shall give him, will become in him a fountain of water springing up into eternal life"* – John 4:13-14. Jesus of course was not speaking of natural water but spiritual water which comes through believing in Him.

How can you inherit eternal life?

Eternal life is something you cannot inherit because of your merit or lifestyle. It is not passed on to you just because your parents may have made it to heaven, or because you have earned it through your good works.

I was in the gym the other day and a lady around my age who knows I am a minister said to me *"Terry, what do you think will happen to me after I die?"* I replied saying *"I hope you will go to Heaven."* She immediately reacted and said, *"No way, heaven is only for GOOD people".* This led to an interesting discussion on how you get to heaven.

A rich young ruler came to Jesus in Matthew 19:16-22 and said to Him **"Good Teacher, what GOOD thing, shall I do that I might inherit eternal life?"** What a great question to ask Jesus. But he is convinced that there is something GOOD he can do to earn eternal life. Jesus went on to say **"Why do you call me GOOD? No one is GOOD, but One, that is God."**

Does this mean that Jesus was not good, of course not He was God in the flesh anyway? No, He was making a point. No matter how good you may be it is not the answer to securing eternal life and getting to Heaven. Jesus implies he could try keeping the commandments. To which the man says he had already kept them. The man then said to Jesus *"What MORE can I DO."* Reading between the lines the answer Jesus gave may have meant if you want perfection, (*go sell what you have and come and follow me*). At that point, the man went on his way, because, he had great possessions.

Jesus went on describing, how hard it was for a rich man, to enter the kingdom of God. He was implying that their riches may get in the way of them wanting to follow Him. But the answer is simple, anyone can be saved, even the rich can be saved, it is by grace that we are saved through faith in Christ.

Some years ago we were involved in an evangelistic program called 'Evangelism Explosion'. It was a door-knock survey. We would knock on doors and ask people to do a religious survey, asking them several questions leading up to the final question which was *"If you were to die today, and stood before God, and He said to you "Why should I let you into heaven, what would you say?"* For memory about 9 out of 10 people would say, because I have lived a GOOD life, or I have done nothing really bad. They were convinced that leading a GOOD life would get them into Heaven. Just like the rich young ruler, who was convinced that he could have eternal life by doing something GOOD to inherit it.

Some things that seem good - may not be good

Something that seems good is not always good. In Genesis 3:6. We read that *"Eve saw that the fruit was GOOD for food, PLEASANT to the eyes and DESIRABLE to make one wise".* The problem was that God had said it was not to be eaten because if you do you shall die. What seemed to be good to her, was used by Satan to deceive her into eating what was forbidden fruit.

So she disobeyed God to partake of something that appeared to be good. The result was because of her disobedience, the human race now faces the death penalty. *"There is a way that seems right to a man, but its end is the way of death"* – Proverbs 14:12.

You can be deceived today by all sorts of things that seem to be good. For example, all the deceptive scams and scammers who are ready to rip you off. They all seem good but are far from being good.

It is not our goodness that saves us from our sins. It is the goodness of God that leads us to repentance. *"Or do you despise the riches of His goodness, forbearance, and longsuffering, not knowing that the goodness of God leads you to repentance?"*– Romans 2:4.

Grace and faith

Technically, there will be no good people in heaven, only sinners saved by grace.

I was going on my usual walk, where I go past some Jehovah's Witnesses, who often set up their stand with literature. I usually walk past them, but decided to stop one day and ask them, how I could gain eternal life, and get to heaven. I knew what they would say, and they did not disappoint me.

They said you have to become one of the 144,000 that are mentioned in the book of Revelation. I asked, how, I could become one of them. They said by your good works. To which, I replied, *"But the bible says"*, ***"For by grace you have been saved through faith, and that not of yourselves; it is the gift of God."*** – Ephesians 2:8. Which they ignored and said, "God must judge you according to your good works to see if you will make it to heaven".

They could not understand how someone could be saved by grace and through faith without good works. Although good works are still to be commended, because when it comes to rewards, we will be rewarded for our good works, but good works alone will not save us. Salvation is a gift to be received by faith in Christ.

Believe and be born again

Nicodemus, a religious leader of the Jews, came to Jesus and said to Him, ***"Rabbi, we know that you are a teacher come from God; for no one can do these signs that you do unless God is with him."*** Jesus answered and said to him, ***"Most assuredly, I say to you, unless one is born again, he cannot see the Kingdom of God."*** – John 3:3.

I think Jesus was concerned that Nicodemus lacked understanding and only had head knowledge, and tried to figure it out with his mind rather than it being a revelation to him by the Spirit. Jesus said to him, ***"That which is born of the flesh is flesh, and that which is born of the Spirit is spirit"***.

Jesus then later challenges him by asking *"Are you the teacher of Israel, and do not know these things?"* – John 3:6-10. Then of course, in the same discourse, we have that great scripture in John 3:16. *"For God so loved the world that He gave his only begotten Son, that whoever believes in Him should not perish but have everlasting life."*

Assurance of salvation

I have had older people in their twilight years begin to doubt their salvation, and say to me, how can I be sure that I am saved and have eternal life? My answer is the same as the answer Jesus gave the devil when He was tempted to doubt God. The answer is "It is written"

I usually then turn them to scriptures like 1 John 5:11-13 *"God has given us eternal life, and this life is in His Son. He who has the Son has life; he who does not have the Son of God does not have life. These things I have WRITTEN to you who believe in the name of the Son of God, that you may KNOW that you have eternal life."* This is more than a feeling it is a fact for it is written.

Having established how we can now find eternal life, I would like to explore in the next chapters what eternity is going to look like, and what we can look forward to with great joy.

Chapter 15

What will Heaven look like?

When we think about Heaven we can begin to imagine all sorts of things. Will we be floating around the clouds playing on harps? Will it be like one long church service? Will we be bored with nothing to do?

I have admired the beauty of this earth in several countries, especially in Papua New Guinea with its outstanding rugged mountain ranges. But for me, Australia takes some beating. I remember when I was younger exploring the beautiful Grampian Mountain Range near my home town of Horsham in Victoria and thinking to myself *"It doesn't get any better than this"*. But it does! It is called Heaven, which according to scripture far surpasses anything we shall ever see here on Earth. We can never comprehend the splendour and the beauty of Heaven. However, the bible gives us a foretaste of what to expect.

175

A real paradise

We live on the Gold Coast which boasts of being a Surfer's Paradise. That is true, but as nice as it is it can never be compared to Heaven.

The apostle Paul was caught up at one stage to 'Paradise' and saw the splendour of heaven and heard things that amazed him that he was even forbidden to share. *"And I know that this man was caught up into Paradise, whether in the body or away from the body I do not know, God knows. And he heard utterances beyond the power of man to put into words, which man is not permitted to utter"* – 2 Corinthians 12:3-4 (AMP). Whatever he saw and heard must have been amazing. It appears that God does not want to reveal everything. He seems to have a few surprises waiting for us.

I remember my mother in her twilight years before she passed on would say *"Terry tell me all about Heaven – what will it be like? Read to me from the bible."* I did the best I could and you could tell she was greatly blessed and was more at peace when I read to her. It was a great tonic for her soul.

I do not want to make light of Heaven but I heard a joke I can't resist telling. *"A new convert, a keen cricketer was trying to find out what Heaven would be like. So he asked the pastor "Do they play cricket in Heaven?"* The pastor said, *"I will ask God and let you know next Sunday."* The following Sunday the keen cricketer asked the pastor, *"What did God say?* The pastor said, *"Well there is good news, and there is bad news." "The good news is, yes, they do play cricket in Heaven". "The bad news is, that you are opening the batting next Saturday."*

Check it out

If you were going to move to a city in another state or country, you would do some research to find out what you could about that city or country. This led me to do a study, to find out from the scriptures more information on what Heaven is going to look like. Although there is not a lot of detail, I was surprised to find several scriptures that brought joy to my heart.

We also have books and testimonies, of some people who have been pronounced dead and visited Heaven and have then been sent back to Earth again to give us an account of what they have seen and heard. Many of these accounts correspond to the bible.

An amazing environment

There is a lot of concern about our environment here on Earth today. Some of the things on top of the world agenda are issues like climate change and its effects on the earth. Other concerns are deforestation, rapid population growth, food production and distribution, global warming, depletion of the ozone layer, acid precipitation, and ocean and air pollution. All this indicates that the earth could be in big trouble in the future.

Heaven is the place to be in the future. It has an amazing environment. There is a perfect city, with a perfect climate. *"The City had no need of the sun or of the moon to shine in it, for the glory of God illuminated it. The Lamb is its light."* Imagine that no more storms, floods, cyclones, tornadoes or climate change issues.

It is also a place where we enjoy perfect health. *"God himself will be with them and be their God. And will wipe away every tear from their eyes; there shall be no more death, nor sorrow, nor crying. There shall be no more pain, for the former things have passed away."* – Revelation 21:23, 3-4.

No more disabilities, no more pain, pills or medication, no more death, or sorrow. Sounds like a great place to be with no more earthly worries, a place where we enjoy a fit and healthy lifestyle.

Your eternal home

There is a worldwide housing crisis today. Some years ago we thought homelessness was only found in third-world countries. But not anymore. The cost of living, and a housing shortage, are driving a surging demand for homeless support. A new analysis by 'Homeless Australians' has found that financial difficulties and housing affordability stress are skyrocketing. Statistics reveal that every night, roughly 1 in 200 Australians find themselves without a safe, secure, or affordable place to sleep.

The basic home is our foundation for safety and security. Access to safe and secure housing is one of the most basic human rights. I see homeless people almost every day somewhere on the beautiful, affluent Gold Coast.

In eternity we have a home prepared for us. *"In my Father's house are many mansions; if it were not so I would have told you. I go to prepare a place for you"*

– John 14:2. We have an eternal home prepared for us, and it's free – it's a part of our salvation package that we have as believers in Christ.

No more rent, no more mortgages, no more rates, no more maintenance. What a blessing, to think we have this fringe benefit, along with the free gift of salvation in Christ. We are not told exactly what that home will look like, but we can be sure it will be beautiful because it is a part of Heaven.

No more bad relationships

There will be no more bad or hurtful relationships. No more pride or jealousy, no more bitterness or resentments, no more revenge or paybacks. No more scammers, no more people out to deceive us, or rip us off. *"Do not be deceived; evil company corrupts good habits"* – 1 Corinthians 15:33.

There will be no evil company to keep, only sinners saved by grace, and transformed into the image of Christ.

Awesome company

We will be surrounded by some awesome company in Heaven. Of course, everything will revolve around Christ and His throne. Christ will sit on the throne and will be worshipped, as the Lamb that was slain. There will be a great host worshipping around the throne. What an awesome sight! *"Then I looked, and heard the voice of many angels around the throne, the living creatures, and the elders; and the number of them was ten thousand times ten thousand, and thousands of thousands"* – Rev 5:11.

Not to mention all the saints and heroes of faith mentioned in the bible, our departed loved ones, our family, our relatives, and our friends, including those we have led to the Lord.

Will we be married in Heaven?

This is a good question and one I am often asked. It is especially applicable to those who have been married several times and wonder who they will end up with in Heaven.

Well, thankfully Jesus answered this question. The Sadducees asked Jesus *"If a woman has had seven husbands and they all die, and then she dies, which one, will she be married to in Heaven? Jesus said you are mistaken for in the resurrection they neither marry nor are given in marriage but are like the angels of God in Heaven"* – Matthew 22:23-33.

My wife does not like this scripture because she knows I love her and thinks I spoil her, and she wants it to go on for eternity in heaven. However, I'm sure we will be able to spend time together. I guess our desires will be somewhat different if we are going to be like the angels.

I remember one of our bible college lecturers being asked this question. He said as much as he loved his wife he could not imagine being married to her for eternity. I hope it never got back to her. Maybe some people with difficult marriages think it is a great thing.

What will Heaven look like?

What will we be doing?

I am sure that we will not be bored. There will be plenty of exciting things to do.

We have been forced to work hard here on Earth because of the fall. We read in Genesis 3:17-19. *"Cursed is the ground for your sake; in toil, you shall eat of it all the days of your life... in the sweat of your face you will eat bread till you return to the ground."*

What can we look forward to in Heaven? There will be no more sweat or hard labour. No, I do not think we will be floating around on clouds playing on harps, (maybe on our day off).

Not a lot of detail is given as to what we will be doing, but it would seem as though we will be involved in many enjoyable activities.

Here is an outline of some events that will be happening at some stage in Heaven-

- **The Wedding Supper of the Lamb**
  "Blessed are those who are invited to the Wedding Supper of the Lamb" – Rev. 19:7-9.
  Maybe there will be other celebrations as well.

- **Worshipping the Lamb that was slain**
  "Blessing and honour and glory and power be to Him who sits on the throne and to the Lamb forever and ever" – Rev. 5:1.

181

- **We will see him face to face**

  "For now we see in a mirror dimly, but then face to face" – 1 Cor. 13:12.

- **Reunions and fellowship**

  Meeting loved ones and fellowshipping with all the Saints – 1 Cor. 15.

- **Answers to Biblical questions**

  "For we know in part and prophecy in part. But when that which is perfect has come, then that which is in part shall be done away" – 1 Cor13:10

- **Serving the Lord**

  "...and His servants will serve Him" – Rev 22:3.

- **Ruling and reigning with Christ**

  "...and will reign with Him" – Rev 5:10.

Rewards for service

We should not forget that Heaven will also be a place where we receive our reward for our service here on Earth. *"And behold I am coming quickly, and My reward is with Me, to give to everyone according to his works".* – Revelation 22:12. All believers will receive their just reward.

I will never forget the vision I had not long after I was saved and I felt God was calling me to be a pastor. I believe

God showed me what a pastor's reward would be.

I saw in the Spirit an image of Jesus standing above the platform at a Christian conference in Adelaide. His image was like bright shining Gold with a shepherd's crook in one hand, a set of scales in the other, and a glorious golden crown upon His head. I did not fully understand what I was seeing at the time (as far as I know nobody else saw Him). I eventually found an appropriate reference to what I saw in the Spirit. *"Shepherd the flock of God which is among you...and when the Chief Shepherd appears you will receive the crown of glory that does not fade away"* – 1 Peter 5:2-4. I believe *'the crown of glory'*, (whatever that may be) is a part of the reward pastors (shepherds) will receive. All believers will be rewarded for their own works and service.

A new Heaven and a new Earth

There are indications in Revelation and Isaiah that our final destination will be a new Earth, on which Heaven descends. *"Now I saw a new Heaven and a new Earth, for the first Heaven and the first Earth had passed away."* – Revelation 21:1.

I like to think of Heaven as a real tangible place, maybe like a new perfect version of Earth. Both a literal place and a spiritual place. We will all have new immortal bodies. Not like disembodied spirits but will be able to taste, touch, feel, see and hear as we do now. (Maybe there will be golf courses after all).

Whatever you anticipate or think about as possibilities for

Heaven, it is bound to be better. This scripture may also refer to Heaven. *"But it is written; Eye has not seen, nor ear heard, nor have entered into the heart of man the things which God has prepared for those who love Him"* – 1 Corinthians 2:9. Whatever God has prepared for us, it will be an amazing place.

Knowing more about Heaven is reassuring for me and I hope you feel the same way. Although we only have a glimpse of what it will be like, we will be serving Him, with great joy and gladness of heart.

This is surely something to rejoice about and look forward to as we enter our twilight years.

Chapter 16

Your resurrection body

As we enter our twilight years, and our bodies become frail we can look forward to one day having a resurrection body. Not that we are in a hurry to get it. The Bible indicates that our resurrection body will be glorious, it will be invincible, free from pain and decay, and never to die again.

Some people over the years have doubted the idea of a resurrection, going way back to the Sadducees in the days of Jesus. However, the Bible is very clear on the matter. So much so that it even states that if Christ did not rise from the dead our faith is in vain.

The credibility of Christianity hangs on the fact of the resurrection of the dead. *"For if the dead do not rise, then Christ is not risen, your faith is futile; you are still in your sin"* – 1 Corinthians 15:16-17.

Hard to imagine

Can you imagine what your resurrection body will look like? I know one skinny little preacher who said he has put his order in for a taller more muscular body. But I'm not sure that it works that way. It will be similar in looks to our natural body, as we will be able to recognize one another, but vastly different in substance. One thing is for sure – you will look great!

We marvel at the indestructible body of 'Superman' in the movies and the incredible feats that he can accomplish. Yet it would appear that our resurrection body will be powerful, not weakened by kryptonite, and would be able to outdo him.

We are not being raised to die again

When we speak of our resurrection body we should not associate our resurrection body with the story of Jesus raising Lazarus from the dead. Martha said to Jesus, *"Lord if only you had been here, my brother would not have died."*....Jesus said to her, *"Your brother will rise again"*. Martha said to him *"I know that he will rise again in the resurrection at the last day."* Jesus said to her, *"I am the resurrection and the life. He who believes in Me, though he may die, he shall live. And whoever lives and believes in Me shall never die. Do you believe this?"* – John 11:21 & 23-26.

Yes, she did believe this, and so do I, and so should you! What a wonderful promise and reassurance we have from Jesus. He went on to raise Lazarus from the dead. However, when Jesus raised Lazarus from the dead he was still in his old mortal body and would have died again at a later date. So our resurrection body is not the body we have now coming back to life in our present form. Even if we had the faith to raise the dead, they are still going to die again.

Our attempt to raise the dead

When we were on the mission field in Port Moresby there was a knock on the door one morning. When I opened the door, four national pastors were standing there. They said they would like me to come and pray for a brother who had died yesterday. I asked where he was, and they said in the van out the front of your house. So I went out and we began to pray hoping to raise him from the dead.

As we prayed we were looking for the flicker of an eyelid or some sign of life. There was none. Maybe we did not have the faith to raise him from the dead. But one by one we felt he wanted to stay in heaven and did not want to come back. But I was very disappointed that we could not raise him from the dead.

Smith Wigglesworth

I had read about Smith Wigglesworth and how it was thought that he raised 14 people from the dead during his ministry. I have no idea how accurate that is. He had a powerful evangelistic healing ministry and saw countless miracles. He used to say *"The Acts of the Apostles were written because the Apostles acted"*. He was a humble man, a plumber by trade. His life changed dramatically after he was baptised in the Holy Spirit at 48 years of age.

It is said that on one occasion he raised his wife Polly from the dead, but she wanted to go back to heaven, so he let her go. Another time it is said that he propped a dead man up in a corner and told him to walk in Jesus' name. Nothing happened, so he persevered, and the third time he told the man to walk he did.

What incredible faith. However, the point is that all of these people that he raised from the dead would eventually die again.

Indwelling resurrection life

According to the scripture, we have a measure of resurrection life dwelling within us now, *"But if the Spirit of Him who raised Jesus from the dead dwells in you, He who raised Christ from the dead will also give life to your mortal bodies through His Spirit who dwells in you"* – Romans 8:11.

I know one pastor who when he was not feeling well would apply this scripture by refusing to let the condition get the better of him by claiming the resurrection life that raised Christ would quicken his mortal body and restore strength and heal him. He lived to over 100, so I guess it worked for him.

I don't know why, and I do not want to be disrespectful, but the above scripture referring to resurrection life in us now reminds me of being able to drink one of those energy drinks that can fire up your electrolytes and keep you hydrated. Anyway, it is something to think about.

Paul answers the question – How are the dead raised?

The Apostle Paul, speaking of the resurrection, asks the question. *"How are the dead raised up and with what body do they come?"* – 1 Corinthians 15:35. He goes on to answer his question, by giving us some insights as to what will happen, and how we will look in our resurrection body.

Paul tells us that first, our natural body must die. This reminds me of a joke. A Sunday school teacher was asking her class *"How can we get to Heaven?"* She said, *"What if I give a lot of money will I get to Heaven?"* The class yells, *"NO!"* Then she said, *"What if I am a good person will I get to Heaven?"* The class yells, *"NO!"* Finally, she said, *"What if I help a lot of people?"* Again the class yells, *"NO!"* Then little Johnny down the back yells out *"I know how you can get to Heaven"*. *"First you have to die."* Yes, little Johnny was right. To get our resurrection body we first have to die.

It would seem that our spirit will go to Heaven immediately when we die in whatever form or shape that may be in, to be later followed on resurrection day by our promised resurrection body that will be with us throughout eternity.

The resurrection process

I will outline how Paul explains the resurrection process and what it will look like, as he does in some detail in 1 Corinthians 15:35-49.

1. Our natural body dies and is sown into the ground like

a seed, but raised in a different form.

2. It is sown as a terrestrial body (earthly). It is raised as a celestial body (heavenly).

3. The terrestrial body has a glory like the Moon. The celestial body has a glory like the Sun. They are vastly different.

4. Our natural body is sown in corruption (it will decay). But it will be raised in incorruption (it will be immortal).

5. It is sown a natural body like Adam. It is raised a spiritual body like Christ.

When Christ returns

Paul encourages us not to be like people who have no hope, but to be comforted by the fact that there will be a great resurrection when Christ appears and returns to this earth with all the saints that have already passed on.

"For the Lord, Himself will descend from Heaven with a shout with the voice of an archangel, and with the trumpet of God. And the dead in Christ will rise first. Then we who are alive and remain shall be caught up together with them in the clouds to meet the Lord in the air. And thus we shall always be with the Lord. Therefore comfort one another with these words." – 1 Thessalonians 4:16-18.

We have not talked about the return of Christ and that great event that is yet to happen. It will take place but we are not told just when. What an incredible day that will be for all believers of all time.

We are told to comfort one another with these words. What a wonderful reunion we have marked sometime in the future, on the heavenly calendar.

The resurrection body of Christ

What was the resurrection body of Christ like? Several scriptures leave me a little intrigued. *"Jesus stood in the midst of them, and said to them "Peace to you". But they were terrified and frightened and supposed they had seen a spirit. And He said to them, "Why are you troubled? And why do doubts arise in your hearts? "Behold My hands and My feet, that it is I Myself". "Handle Me and see, for a spirit does not have flesh and bones as you see I have." ....He said to them, "Have you any food here". "So they gave Him some broiled fish and some honeycomb. And He took it and ate it in their presence"* – Luke 24:36-39 & 41-43.

We learn from this scripture that Jesus' resurrected body was recognisable and very much in human form. But we also realise that a normal body of flesh and bones would have had trouble walking through a wall, (in the gospel of John it says the doors were shut indicating Jesus just suddenly appeared in their midst). Maybe the flesh and bones were of a different substance or could transform somehow into a spiritual form to enable Him to walk through a wall. Then to complicate things He asked for food and ate it.

I doubt that our resurrection bodies will need food to survive, but I find it comforting to know he was able to eat. If we can eat I do not think we will have any weight problems. Maybe there are coffee shops in Heaven after all.

A Biblical description of your resurrection body

The following bible verses describe your resurrection body as follows –

1. **A Christ-like bod**y – *"We know that when He is revealed we shall be like Him."* – 1 John 3:2.

2. **A tangible Body** – *"Reach your finger here, and look at my hands; and reach your hand here, and put it into my side."* – John 20:27.

3. **A God-designed body** – *"But God gives us a body as He pleases."* – 1 Corinthians 15:38.

4. **A powerful body** – *"It is sown in weakness, it is raised in power."* – 1 Corinthians 15:43.

5. **Angel-like** – *"In the resurrection they neither marry nor are given in marriage, but are like the angels in Heaven."* – Matthew 22:30.

6. **A spiritual body** – *"It is raised a spiritual body."* – 1 Corinthians 15:44.

7. **An immortal and incorruptible body** – *"What is raised is imperishable"* – 1 Corinthians 15:42.

Overall Summary

Our old physical body will be left behind; our new spiritual body will be raised perfectly suited to be with the Lord in Heaven forever.

1. **It can never be destroyed**
   It is immortal and eternal, it will never be disabled, get sick, or suffer from pain. (No more doctors or pills).

2. **It will be recognizable**
   Others will be able to recognize us and we will be able to recognize them. (No need to shave or wear makeup or have haircuts)

3. **It will be incredible**
   Jesus suddenly appeared and disappeared. It will be indestructible (No need for a car or public transport).

I hope you find these thoughts comforting and encouraging, as you enter your twilight years. They bring joy to my heart, knowing that one day I will have a resurrection body and Heaven is my final destination. I hope you feel the same way.

Chapter 17

Are you ready for Heaven?

How do you know if you are ready for Heaven? What is going to happen to you after your twilight years have expired? It is one thing to know about Heaven; it is another thing to believe in your heart, by faith, that you are ready.

Without Christ, nobody is ready or fit for Heaven. No one deserves to go to Heaven – it is not through your good deeds or your lifestyle that you will get to Heaven. None of us will ever measure up. *"All have sinned and fall short of the glory of God"* – Romans 3:23. It is only by the grace of God that anybody makes it.

Anne Ross Cousin wrote a hymn with the first two lines declaring, 'The sands of time are sinking – 'The dawn of Heaven breaks'. Once we enter our twilight years the sands of time are sinking for us, but the good news is that the dawn

195

of heaven breaks. Once our life on earth is finished we have the assurance that the door of heaven will open to welcome us to enter into another exciting adventure.

Again I do not want to be disrespectful but I am reminded of a joke about a couple on Earth who had a wonderful marriage. Unfortunately, the wife became ill and eventually died. She went to Heaven and was met by Peter at the Pearly Gates. He asked her to spell one word for him to open the gate. The word was 'love,' so she spelled it and entered heaven. A few years later Peter asked her to fulfill his duty at the gate for a week while he had a break. She remembered that people had to spell the word 'love' to get in. After a few days at the gate, who should appear but her husband. She asked how he survived without her and he said, *"Really well"*, *"I got together with that young nurse that was looking after you when you were sick"*. *"We traveled around the world, spent all our savings, and had a marvelous time."* Then he asked, *"Are you going to open the gate for me?"* She replied, *"You have to spell one word."* *"What is it?"* She said, *"Czechoslovakia."*

Is it possible for you to make it?

You might be thinking to yourself, how can a sinner, a guilty and shameful failure like me be accepted by a good and perfect and Holy God? How can that be? That is answered by the power of the gospel (good news) which declares that you are saved by grace through faith in Christ who died on the cross and shed His blood to cleanse you from all your sin and to set you free from all the condemnation that the devil would throw at you.

Jesus warns us to be ready. *"Therefore you also be ready, for the Son of Man is coming at an hour you do not expect"* – Matthew 24:44. I know this is in the context of the second coming of Christ. But I would take the liberty of using it as a warning for us to be ready to meet Jesus when we die, for we are only a heartbeat away from eternity, and we have no idea when that might be.

What value do you place on your soul? Your soul is going to live on forever throughout all eternity, either in Heaven or in Hell. Jesus said, *"For what profit is it for a man if he gains the whole world, and loses his own soul? Or what will a man give in exchange for his soul"* – Matthew 16:26. There is nothing you can exchange for your soul.

You cannot buy your way to Heaven. Surely nobody in their right mind wants to lose their soul, and as a result, spend eternity in Hell. In terms of value, our soul is more valuable than all the wealth and earthly possessions we may gain here on earth. They will all perish but our soul lives on forever.

God steps in to save us

God has done an amazing thing. It is hard for us to fully understand it. He stepped down from His throne in heaven and came into this earth as a baby. *"For there is born to you this day in the City of David a Saviour who is Christ the Lord. "And this will be a sign to you. You will find a Babe wrapped in swaddling cloth's lying in a manger"*. – Luke 2:10-12.

This is called the 'Incarnation of Christ' something we

197

celebrate and sing about every Christmas. We often see those lovely nativity scenes depicting this story. But have you ever seriously thought about the wonder of this?

It is greater than any of the 'Seven Wonders of the World'. To think that Almighty God would step down from His throne in Heaven and come to us as vulnerable as a baby. Who as a baby had to be fed, toilet trained, learn to walk and talk, experience the full spectrum of human emotions, be educated, and work for a living before His public ministry began. This is amazing! I marvel at this, and to think He did this to save sinners like you and me. Surely this is the amazing Grace of God.

The apostle John puts it this way. *"In the beginning was the Word and the Word was with God, and the Word was God."…. "And the Word became flesh and dwelt among us, and we beheld His glory, as of the only begotten of the Father, full of grace and truth."* – John 1:1 & 14.

Yes, the Word was God and became flesh (Jesus) and dwelt among us. Amazing!

Salvation is a gift

We live in a world of inflation. The cost of everything seems to be rapidly increasing as the years unfold. The only thing that is not inflating is the gift of salvation. It is, and always will be, completely free for all those who seek it.

We read in Romans 6:23 *"For the wages of sin is death,*

but the gift of God is eternal life in Christ Jesus our Lord." We see that the wages of sin are death. We have all sinned so we are all in big trouble. But the good news is that the gift of God is eternal life, because of Christ. Please note this is a gift from God – it is something, we do not deserve, and can never earn through our good works. Christ has set us free from eternal damnation and has given us the gift of eternal life.

What we need to do is believe, and repent, which means we need to decide to turn away from our sins, and turn to Christ, asking Him to forgive us and come into our life. This means a change of direction in our life. So to become a Christian we need to believe. *"God so loved the world that He gave us His only begotten Son, that whoever believes in Him should not perish but have everlasting life"* – John 3:16. Evangelist Billy Graham once explained this process by preaching *"Change your mind [repent] and He will change your heart."*

This is the grace of God being extended to us *"For by grace you have been saved through faith, and that not of yourselves; it is the gift of God, not of works lest anyone should boast."* – Ephesians 2:8.

So the bible re-affirms that salvation has nothing to do with us or our works. God took the initiative by sending Jesus to shed his blood on the cross for the forgiveness of our sins. God first loved us. He loves you 'so' much that sent Jesus to become the sacrificial lamb for your sins.

If the thief on the cross can make it - so can you!

Think about it! Two thieves were being crucified with Jesus and they were both mocking Jesus at one stage. Then one of them at the last minute must have changed his mind and said to Jesus, *"Lord remember me when you come into your Kingdom"*. And Jesus said to him, *"I say to you, today you will be with Me in Paradise"*. – Luke 23:42-43.

I can imagine this thief being questioned from a theological point of view by some when he arrived in Paradise. *"How come you made it?"* *"Did you attend the synagogue regularly?"* *"Do you know the scriptures?"* He probably would have been a little confused. Then they would have asked, *"Well, why are you here?"* His answer would have been, *"I'm not sure, all I know is the man called Jesus said I could come. "I'm here because of Him"*. This is the amazing grace of God in action.

However, the thief on the cross must have been displaying some kind of faith, whether out of desperation or hope, by asking the Lord to remember him when He entered His kingdom.

It is highly unlikely that he had any theological understanding of what was happening at the time. He does not appear to be a religious man. How then was it possible for him to make it to Heaven? I will explain this in the next section

The precious blood of Jesus

The only reason the thief on the cross made it was because

of the precious blood of Jesus. *"Knowing that you were not redeemed with corruptible things...but with the precious blood of Christ, as a lamb without blemish and without spot".* – 1 Peter 1:18-19.

The thief would have seen the blood-stained body of Jesus, but would not have realised how precious that blood was to become, not only for him but for the whole human race.

This is at the heart of the gospel. It is the message that will get you to Heaven. It is the only reason any of us will make it

That Guy

I was at my son's place recently, and Ruth, his wife showed me a book they were reading. Its title was 'How to talk about Jesus without being 'THAT GUY'. The theme of the book is how to share your faith with others without having a reputation of being 'that guy' who is a pain in the neck because he is always talking about Jesus and is inclined to put people off.

I agree and think there is a lot of wisdom in that thought. I'm sure we have all come across 'that guy' at some stage. At the risk of being 'that guy' this once, may I remind you, how important it is to be ready to meet Jesus! If you want to make sure you are ready then this is your opportunity to do something about it.

If that is you, I would like you to read this scripture before I pray for you. *"If you confess with your mouth the Lord Jesus and believe in your heart that God has raised Him from the dead, you will be saved. For with the heart, one believes unto righteousness, and with the mouth, confession is made unto salvation"* – Romans 10:9-10.

Are you ready to believe in your heart, and confess with your mouth, declaring Christ as your Saviour? Then if you want to, I will now lead you in prayer.

"Lord I come to you now, asking for your forgiveness for all my sins. Come into my life, and make me a new person. I believe in my heart right now and confess with my mouth that you are my Saviour and Lord."

If you prayed that simple prayer, congratulations, you are now a child of God, and ready for Heaven.

I would encourage you to find a good church where they preach the word of God so you can grow and mature as a Christian.

I thank you for reading this book, and I pray that it will have helped you in many areas of your life, and make you more able to fully appreciate and enjoy your twilight years. †

www.ingramcontent.com/pod-product-compliance
Lightning Source LLC
Chambersburg PA
CBHW021904020426
42334CB00013B/481